PRAISE FOR *INSTANT RECESS*

"Dr. Toni (Antronette) Yancey has influenced and impacted community health and fitness in a number of profound ways! Her book is a must-read for anyone interested in living a longer, healthier, and more fulfilling life. Recently, at the First AME Church of Los Angeles, we incorporated a quick but effective fitness interlude into all three of our Sunday worship services. The enthusiastic response from our congregation was tremendous! Thank you, Dr. Yancey, for waking us up to the dangers of our sedentary lives and for awakening our desire to get into better physical shape."

> REV. DR. JOHN & DENISE HUNTER, Pastor and First Lady of First AME Church of Los Angeles, the White House–designated local lead agency for Michelle Obama's Let's Move initiative in L.A.

"A thoughtful and innovative approach to community-wide physical activity from a lay person's perspective. This book is well grounded in scientific evidence that is also contextualized in simple examples and in real life experiences people will be able to relate to."

> ADRIAN BAUMAN, Professor of Public Health, University of Sydney

Instant Recess

BUILDING A FIT NATION
10 MINUTES AT A TIME

TONI YANCEY, MD, MPH

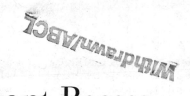

UNIVERSITY OF CALIFORNIA PRESS
Berkeley   Los Angeles   London

University of California Press, one of the most distinguished university presses in the United States, enriches lives around the world by advancing scholarship in the humanities, social sciences, and natural sciences. Its activities are supported by the UC Press Foundation and by philanthropic contributions from individuals and institutions. For more information, visit www.ucpress.edu.

University of California Press
Berkeley and Los Angeles, California

University of California Press, Ltd.
London, England

Library of Congress Cataloging-in-Publication Data
    Yancey, Antronette K.
       Instant recess : building a fit nation 10 minutes at a time /
    Toni Yancey.
       p. ; cm.
       Includes bibliographical references and index.
       ISBN 978-0-520-26375-8 (cloth : alk. paper) —
       ISBN 978-0-520-26376-5 (pbk. : alk. paper)
       1. Health promotion—United States.   2. Physical fitness—United
    States.   3. Exercise—United States.   I. Title.
       [DNLM: 1. Physical Fitness—United States.   2. Exercise—
    United States.   3. Health Promotion—methods—United States.
    4. Obesity—prevention & control—United States. QT 255 Y21i 2010]
    RA427.8.Y35   2010
    613.0973—dc22   2010024933

Manufactured in the United States of America

19 18 17 16 15 14 13 12 11 10
10 9 8 7 6 5 4 3 2 1

This book is printed on Cascades Enviro 100, a 100% post consumer waste, recycled, de-inked fiber. FSC recycled certified and processed chlorine free. It is acid free, Ecologo certified, and manufactured by BioGas energy.

To my granddaughter, Anaïs Ximena Strong Orozco,
on whom the sun rises and sets, and who is one of the
best things that ever happened to me; her mother,
Kanitra, one of the most genuine and good-hearted
human beings I know; her father, Oscar, who has
my grandfather's name and gentle spirit; and her
grandmother, Darlene, the love of my life.

Contents

Preface   ix

Acknowledgments   xi

Abstract   xiii

Introduction   1

A bleak future · What's *recess* got to do with it? · The mess we've
created · Digging ourselves out! · Why a book? · Why this
idea? · Why this book? · *Instant Recess* . . . in a nutshell

1   The High Price of a Sedentary America and the Challenge of
    Getting Society Moving   22

The lure of the couch is costing us and killing us! · The challenge:
The deck is stacked against us! · The science-industrial complex

2   The Benefits of Widespread Physical Activity and
    Opportunities to Move the Needle   54

There's almost nothing exercise *can't* fix—or at least improve on a
bit · The opportunity: A little goes a looong way · So where do we
go from here?

3   The Evolution of an Idea   78
    Who, exactly, is talking? · How I fell in love with public health ·
    A mosaic of lenses · A historical perspective · Launching my life's
    work · An emerging perspective · Inspiration—the art and science
    behind the recess model · Science, like politics, is usually personal

4   The Marketing and Social Marketing of Physical Activity
    and Fitness   108
    Why a marketing perspective? · Evolution of the public face
    of physical activity · Why marketing? Why now? · What we
    did, and why and how we did it · Current activity marketing
    campaigns · Looking to the future: A model for the social
    marketing of *Instant Recess* · The messenger and the medium

5   The Case for the *Instant Recess* Model   140
    The conceptual framework · How does it work? · How can *you*
    make it work? · Is it workable? · How to get it to work in *your*
    organization · Wrapping it up and putting a bow on it

6   *Instant Recess*—What's Good for the Waistline Is Good for
    the Bottom Line!   175
    Does it work? · Dissemination · Intervention spotlight · *Instant
    Recess* Leaves the Nest · Where we're going from here

7   A Glimpse into the Future: How the Recess Model Sparked a
    Physical Activity Movement   219
    Why *Instant Recess* worked · How *Instant Recess* worked · Toward
    a brighter future . . .

    References   241
    About the Author   253
    Index   255

Appendices are available at www.toniyancey.com.

Preface

I feel in my bones, have for a long time, that movers and shakers—literally, athletes and former athletes, dancers, playground hackers, hikers and nature lovers, military types, putterers and fidgeters—will be the catalysts for community-wide fitness promotion. Of course, we're also part of the problem. We're the plurality if not the majority of physical activity researchers and practitioners. We're the ones who are developing the policies and programs that often overlook the fact that others are not as enamored of moving as we are. *Instant Recess* may spark a social movement embracing widespread physical activity participation, and it may not. But action is better than inaction, and we've got the "sharp elbows" to get it done! As I quip in my poem, "Different," in my parents' house,

> "Can't" was a dirty word
> Worse thing you can say to a kid
> Though *I* wouldn't know
> They never said that to *me* . . .*

*Published in *An Old Soul with a Young Spirit: Poetry in the Era of Desegregation Recovery* (Imhotep, 1997) and *Renaissance Woman/Race Woman* (Imhotep, 2001).

And I'm too stubborn to learn that word at this late date. I've also crossed paths with more than my share of divas—some patients, some peers, some who've lent their celebrity to various of my philanthropic causes—whose belief in me broadened my horizons, expanded my possibilities, and validated my ideas and talent—Linda, Nina, Sharon, Karan, Lesa, Denese, Butch, Kim, Nancy, Marq, Rudi, and Phyllis, to name a few. I'm on a mission, but I need help! So I hope this book will mobilize people smarter, more energetic, and better connected than I to do whatever it takes to get society moving, literally!

Acknowledgments

I'm deeply grateful to Danielle, my Head Diva in Charge, whose creativity and doer spirit infuses all of my work; John, for his incredible editing skills and belief in this cause; Naomi, for her patience and expertise in shepherding this project; Linda, for sending Naomi to me; Cindy, Jonathan T., Shiriki, Roshan, Holly, Kristin H., Shawn, Allen, Bobby, Dave, Jeff, Michele, and Kristin B., for embracing the recess concept and trusting me to make it happen; Melicia, Joni, and NiCole, for leveraging their connections to help me make it happen; and Jonathan F. and Les, for encouraging me to systematically test the concept early and often.

My thanks also go to Todd, York, Ruane, Anat, and Bill R. for lending their artistic vision and genius; Mary B. and Gail, for helping me negotiate the "deal"; Bette and Andrea, for stepping in and lending their marketing expertise in the eleventh hour; Bruce and Bonnie, for showing up just when I needed them most; Mary P., Joanne, Octavia, Joyce, Mona, Jammie, Portia, Denise, Carmen B., Lorenzo, Juanita, Candice, Carmen N., Loma, Jaime, Suzanne, and Rebecca, who read the book or portions of it and gave me the benefit of their wisdom; Mark and Eric, for their advice about book publishing and marketing; Mark, Karen, Kate, and Kalicia for their production assistance; my friends and colleagues who provided illustrations for the book, including Jim, Amy, Sue, Tim, and the San Diego Padres, EnviroMedia, Eduardo, and Roberto.

Finally, I thank my students and all of the people representing a host of organizations who have participated in my research studies and taught me a lot of what I know; and all who're inspired to reintegrate a little *Instant Recess* into the routine of the places where they work, learn, play, worship, advocate, network, socialize, or otherwise congregate.

Abstract

The societal benefits of physical activity cannot be fully realized until most people get moving. Physical exertion has been prompted by necessity throughout most of human history and is still considered unappealing in most forms by all but a small minority. To date, however, most activity research and practice is predicated upon increasing active recreation. Despite a forty-year investment in education and counseling, leisure time has become less active, and physical activity levels have plummeted. A different approach is needed, one that is grounded in the cultures and preferences of the sedentary majority. Reintegrating short bouts of enjoyable activity into workplace, school, religious, and social settings in which people congregate for other purposes makes the active choice the easy or default choice—the path of least resistance—and the inactive choice socially undesirable, much as smoking bans catalyzed the tobacco control movement. *Instant Recess* makes the case that what's good for the waistline is good for the bottom line. The book argues that when leaders are persuaded of the substantial return on investment in enhanced worker productivity or student academic performance delivered by implementing *Instant Recess®* breaks, the physical activity promotion movement will gain traction. The collective volition of leaders with a strong incentive to accomplish their organizational aims, rather than individual motivation, will drive the more sweeping societal changes necessary to restore regular activity participation.

Introduction

To most people, Pixar's animated movie *WALL-E* was about two robots trying to find love. But to me, a public health doc, it was a thinly veiled parable of the horrors that humans face if we don't act immediately to solve one of the most pressing public health crises we've ever encountered.

WALL-E's world is the near future, in which robots have taken over all the mundane tasks we used to perform, and humans have evolved into fat blobs with atrophied arms and legs—inactive, unfit, and dangerously complacent and incurious.

This being a Pixar movie, little WALL-E and his love become catalysts for the humans to finally get out of their easy chairs and save themselves, and as the closing credits roll, we see humans, generation by generation, regaining health, mobility, sanity, curiosity, and joie de vivre as they take control of their lives again.

But back here in real life, at the dawn of the second decade of the twenty-first century, there's no Hollywood ending in sight. The latest figures show the average American is very sedentary and out of shape, and most of the rest of the developed world's population is not far behind. The monetary and social costs are already mounting, and our future looks increasingly bleak. If we don't act now, we won't be able to stop that nightmare from becoming a reality.

This book offers a way out, a simple way to arrest the growth of the twin epidemics of sedentariness and obesity and then, through further natural steps, to rebuild a healthy America. It's simple, but it's not easy, because it will take more than a couple of love-struck robots to rescue us. It'll take a concerted effort at all levels of society. But my approach is also designed to ignite a brushfire—an *epidemic*, if you will—of regular, routine, nearly inescapable activity. My research suggests that the changes I'd implement would spread as their success became apparent and as the economic and societal benefits manifested themselves.

Sedentariness is a societal problem, but it's also an individual problem. Take my friend and colleague, for instance . . .

WHAT'S RECESS GOT TO DO WITH IT?

One of my close colleagues for the past twenty years, let's call her Mary— a middle-aged woman of Asian extraction with a powerful job, a great figure, and an only kid safely ensconced at a prestigious university (in other words, someone who should know better)—will tell you flat out, "I hate to exercise! I'd rather just not eat." And in fact, about the only thing she exercises regularly is restraint: when it comes to her diet, she'll often skip dinner to make room—in her calorie count, not her stomach—for dessert.

On rare occasions, Mary allows herself to be dragged out of her office for a lunchtime walk. But she's very clear that the only way she's going to exercise regularly is if she has to trip over it. And, indeed, her motivation comes from her co-workers, friends, and associates. Going on walking meetings with her boss and participating in group exercise breaks during meetings are about as good as it gets. Like a lot of other people, Mary needs social interactions and expectations, mixed with a little peer pressure that's embedded in organizational routine, to be dragged not quite kicking and screaming out of her seat. But in those group breaks, she enjoys moving with her co-workers to old-school rock and disco classics, the way Richard Simmons's groupies do on *Sweatin' with the Oldies*. But Mary and her co-workers are really more like glowin', since most don't come close to breaking a sweat, nor do they have to don any sweats to participate. Matter of fact, back in her soccer mom days, Mary could even be persuaded to take a walk around the field with the other parents during their kids' practice. Left to her own devices, though, she'd be rooted to the bleachers, tapping out proposals or papers or e-mails or memos on her laptop.

Those of us who came of age several decades ago were not socialized to consider most sports or fitness activities feminine or appropriate for girls, and this is still mostly true today. For most women, physical activity serves a purpose in weight control and not much else. So for highly educated white or Asian women, the desire to be thin can be pretty strong motivation to hit the pavement—unless, as it does for Mary, a dose of dietary restraint does the trick. But for women in other ethnic or cultural groups, where there's less pressure to be thin, there's not a lot of impetus to be active. And, in fact, women of color have some of the lowest physical activity levels of any group.

Furthermore, across the board, whether they make minimum wage or the mid-six figures, women tend to prioritize work and family over self-care. In the time they do make for themselves, they prefer the pampering variety that provides immediate gratification—manicures, pedicures, and hairstyling. And that kind of pampering don't come cheap!

Let's get back to Mary. At least she *admits* that she's not particularly motivated to get moving. She's like most other Americans—male, female, rich, poor, black, brown, red, yellow, or white—who pay lip service to the importance of physical activity and even sing the praises of certain types of activities, like walking on the beach or dancing at a party. But they make excuses about not having the time to exercise or being unable to afford a gym membership; they plop down in front of the TV after work instead of walking around the neighborhood and spend Saturdays in the hair salon, not on the tennis courts. What they say and what they do are miles apart.

Mary's the rule, not the exception. The overwhelming majority of people are relatively inactive. Only about one in five meet the minimum Centers for Disease Control and Prevention (CDC) physical activity recommendations, and until the active choice becomes the default choice—the quickest and easiest way to get through the day, the path of least resistance—that's not going to change. Some of you are probably asking yourselves, "So what? Why should we care? If people want to be slugs, why not let 'em?"

Economists are particularly agnostic about these things. Their perspective, in stark contrast to us public health do-gooders, is that people make decisions to allocate their scarce resources like time, energy, and money, in their own best interests, to maximize their own happiness. Economists are purveyors of freedom of choice, free will, life, liberty, and the pursuit of happiness. But it's becoming clearer even to the Alan Greenspans of the world that people are not making the best choices for the public good (reminiscent of the Wall Street thirty-somethings that brought down the financial markets worldwide), and that rampant sedentariness is costing everyone, not just those who choose that lifestyle. When an ambulance picks up a forty-year-old with a first-time heart attack, *your* tax dollars are likely being needlessly wasted. Co-workers who sit for hours on end at work and at home—getting early-onset diabetes, hypertension, or colon cancer—are raising the medical insurance rating for your company and *your* premiums.

But it's also becoming clear that our will is not so free and our choices are not so self-determined: some neighborhoods have a park on every corner, and others have none at all; some people have flex time and on-site fitness facilities at work, while others punch a time clock and have to get permission even to walk to the bathroom; all kids are bombarded by advertising, not only for sugary drinks and fast food, but also for movies, cars, and video games that exercise only the thumbs, before they're cognitively able to distinguish commercial enticements from factual presentations in the classroom. And if childhood habits like brand selection didn't persist into adulthood, corporations wouldn't invest so many marketing dollars in trying to establish them.

THE MESS WE'VE CREATED

In the 1970s, approximately 20 percent of Americans reported engaging in regular leisure time exercise (Sturm 2004). Times have changed, but the needle hasn't budged. About the same percentage of Americans report engaging in regular leisure time physical activity today (ibid.), but *total* physical activity—not exercise* per se—has fallen precipitously since the 1950s and 1960s, commensurate with the growth of private transportation, the suburbanization of America, the proliferation of labor-saving devices, the deterioration of physical education in schools, and the explosion of information technology (Brownson, Boehmer, and Luke 2005). Couch potatoes at home have become "mouse potatoes" at work, sending electronic mail messages to co-workers in the next cubicle.

This really shouldn't be that surprising, given what we know about evolution. Conserving energy is evolutionarily programmed. The energy necessary to dodge predators and forage for food tilted energy imbalance toward starvation for most of human history. Those who survived to pass on their genes were largely the ones who preferred to rest when they weren't chasing their dinner and to gorge themselves when a meal was handy. It wasn't "overconsuming" during the Stone Age—it was smart! That set of genes dictating that we move only when necessary and consume as much fatty and sugary food as possible hasn't changed much. Certainly not in the mere half-century since *obligatory* or *incidental* activity has dropped dramatically, and the variety and accessibility of

---

*Physical activity encompasses all movement of large muscle groups for any purpose, including transportation, work, aesthetic pleasure (such as strolling on the beach), avocation (bird watching, for instance), or fitness. Exercise is a subset of physical activity aimed at improving some component of fitness—body composition, aerobic endurance (heart-lung functioning), muscular strength, flexibility, or muscular endurance.

tasty, cheap, nutrient-poor but widely and seductively marketed foods have exploded. Evolution simply doesn't move that quickly and hasn't caught up with this new reality of human existence.

We can't wait for evolution. Our inordinately high levels of physical inactivity, combined with an overweight rate of two-thirds of US adults, make it critical that we develop approaches to lifestyle change targeting the *majority* of adults, who are both overweight and sedentary. To get specific, at most 25 percent of the population is regularly active at recommended levels, 14 percent is completely sedentary, and 25 percent reports absolutely no physical activity beyond that necessary for daily functioning—that is, walking from the house to the car, from the couch to the fridge, from the bedroom to the bathroom. Or, as the late comedian Joey Adams once quipped, "If it weren't for the distance from the refrigerator to the TV, some of us wouldn't get any exercise at all!" (Of course, that's a bit of an overstatement. There is the upper-body workout from rummaging under the couch cushions to find the remote.) For example, more than 40 percent of Los Angeles County's 10 million adults report fewer than 10 minutes per *week* of continuous physical activity, and these statistics probably overestimate actual activity levels (Yancey, Wold, et al. 2004). Nationally, a study using accelerometers (glorified pedometers, or step counters) instead of self-report surveys, found that US adults total, on average, only 6 to 10 minutes of moderate to vigorous activity daily, and fewer than 5 percent meet CDC activity recommendations (Troiano et al. 2008).

Adding insult to injury, we've essentially abdicated our responsibility for our kids' fitness to corporate America. We've permitted kids to be besieged by commercial appeals for cars, movies, sedentary video games, highly processed nutrient-poor foods and their promotional toys during Saturday morning TV shows, at school, and in neighborhoods. Rates of childhood obesity are rising rapidly, accompanied by declining fitness levels, particularly in lower-income or ethnic minority communities. Obesity rates have tripled among all school-aged children and quadrupled among adolescents, to almost one in five nationally. But in many urban school districts, up to half of children are overweight or obese (Slusser et al. 2005). Latino and black children at birth have nearly

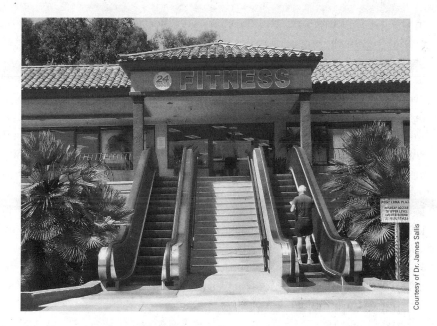

Courtesy of Dr. James Sallis

Figure 1. One wouldn't want to break a sweat on the way to the gym! Obviously, we need to change our compartmentalized notion of exercise and capitalize on any and every opportunity to be active.

a one in two chance of developing diabetes in their lifetime compared with a still-unacceptably high rate of one in four among white children (Narayan et al. 2003).

It gets worse. Even people deemed regularly physically active by the CDC and American College of Sports Medicine—those engaging in 30 minutes of exercise per day at moderate to vigorous intensity on most days of the week—are probably not active enough to maintain a healthy body weight and optimal chronic disease protection. Those 30 minutes a day simply can't replace the exercise we used to get when we weren't "exercising" thirty or more years ago—walking to work or the streetcar, raking leaves and mowing grass, doing indoor household chores, or simply not sitting for hours on end. Especially when we drive around to find the closest parking spot to the gym, take the escalator up to the door, and spend more time altogether in the car than we do in the gym! If anything, as I mentioned earlier, the small proportion of people regularly engaged in leisure time exercise or active recreation has remained the same or grown only a bit—still in the neighborhood of one in four or five. During this period, our waistlines have grown even more. Researchers have already begun to examine the physiology of inactivity, as distinct from the physiology of exercise, arguing that the risk of adverse health and metabolic effects (for example, abnormal cholesterol levels and lower glucose tolerance) from prolonged periods of sitting is independent of, and equal to, the risk of not getting enough exercise (Owen, Bauman, and Brown 2009). For instance, recent studies have found that the number of times people get up and move is linked to their weight, independent of the total number of minutes they spend moving—thinner folks are up and down more often (Hamilton, Hamilton, and Zderic 2007; Mark and Janssen 2009). This has led to calls for changes in the federal activity recommendations to reflect these findings (Hamilton et al. 2008).

DIGGING OURSELVES OUT!

I worked on a committee with a number of colleagues—researchers from many disciplines and regions of the country—to generate the scientific evidence base for the first-ever Physical Activity Guidelines for Americans (Physical Activity Guidelines Advisory Committee 2008). That was in 2008. But the *Dietary* Guidelines for Americans have been released every five years since 1976 (an initiative introduced by a Senate Select Committee headed by George McGovern). Physical activity plays a central role in maintaining, restoring, and enhancing health and well-being, but its role has yet to be fully acknowledged and appreciated. Our committee report underscored that physical activity acts both directly, to protect us against many common chronic conditions, and indirectly, to protect us against chronic disease by helping to prevent weight gain in the first place and to stabilize weight after losing a few pounds. We supported the minimum recommendation of the CDC in 1995 of 30 minutes of at least moderate-intensity physical activity daily for general health,

and highlighted the weight control and other advantages of longer duration and more vigorous activity. However, we also emphasized that there
is no apparent minimum threshold for getting some benefits. In other
words, every minute of activity counts, and the less active you are, the
more you gain from adding a few. But despite a flood of information
documenting its spectrum of benefits and rapid advances in the science
of getting certain individuals to take up activity, the investigation of
how to sustain uptake and promote physical activity across an entire
population is still in its infancy.

We're making good progress in protecting health on some fronts,
and there's an important lesson there. Take smoking. Ten years ago,
the UCLA research team of which I'm a member found that local docs
thought the best way to get smokers to quit was to explain the adverse
health effects of smoking. But, of course, the overwhelming majority
of smokers already know how bad it is for their health, and most have
tried to quit a number of times. Ultimately their success is governed by
elements of their social environment that most don't consciously try to
influence . . . like setting a quit date and publicizing it among family,
friends, and co-workers and finding social outlets to replace the camaraderie of breaks and quiet escapes for a cigarette with other smokers.
Of course, these personal changes act in concert with the diminishing
number of places where smoking is permitted, the rising social disapproval of smoking, the escalation of cigarette prices, and the prohibition
of most cigarette advertising.

Then consider drinking and driving. When I was in medical school
thirty years ago, "one for the road" was the norm. You didn't leave a party
without someone pressing a last drink on you. But Mothers Against
Drunk Driving (MADD) and others helped get rid of that tradition by
showing us the gory and tragic results of drunk driving and pressuring
lawmakers to take action. As societal outrage grew, the alcohol industry
was prompted by the Harvard University Alcohol Project to adopt and
disseminate the now-ubiquitous term *designated driver*. (No matter that
it was mostly to ensure that all but a teetotaling few would be able to
maintain high levels of consumption of their products at social gatherings!) Today, instead of "one for the road," we make it a point to show

our hosts that we're sober when we make our exit from parties. At stake are not only individual consequences (suspension of driving privileges, criminal penalties, and so on) but also liability for hosts and bartenders who knowingly serve intoxicated revelers who are soon-to-be drivers. Traffic-crash death rates attributed to alcohol fell more than 50 percent between 1982 and 2001 (Cummings et al. 2006). And the government is keeping the message from getting stale with new social marketing campaigns such as the public service announcements that ran in the summer of 2009. They featured young and middle-aged handsome, prosperous-appearing white men—a very high-risk population for binge drinking and driving while intoxicated—with cars or motorcycle helmets full of martinis or beer that poured out after they were pulled over by the cops. The tag line, emphasizing the poor chance of escaping detection when stopped, was "over the limit, under arrest."

The take-home message about smoking and booze is now clear to almost everyone: use in moderation. But the message about eating is far from clear, and worse, it's dangerously contradictory. Most overweight people are quite aware of how their condition hurts their lives and their future. Most have dieted frequently. But long-term success in anything is dictated by the sustainability of the changes people make. The personal is bolstered by the social and political. On one hand, the social stigma against obesity is so oppressive that most people say they'd rather have cancer than be fat. But on the other hand, gluttony and nutrient-poor food choices are socially embraced, prompted, and even glorified. It's like a scene from Dante's *Inferno*: obese folks' evolutionarily derived biology tells them to fatten up in case there's a famine, their fellow citizens shun and mock them for being fat, while their physical and social surroundings tempt them mercilessly to gorge themselves.

Commercials masterfully subvert all of our knowledge about what we *should* be doing, in service of what we *want* to do. Food industry scientists are paid the big bucks to design irresistible foods; and marketing agencies, to get people to consume them. That Carl's Jr. TV ad showing a stack of bacon cheeseburgers with the ketchup, guacamole, and mayo spilling down the side and over the cute young skinny guy's shoes makes me want to go out and order a burger, and I'm a public health doc and fitness enthusiast, not even in the targeted market segment for that ad spot . . . plus I don't even eat beef! But nowhere is the triumph of emotion over reason more apparent than in Taco Bell's "Fourthmeal" advertising campaign, the "melty/crunchy/spicy/grilled meal between dinner and breakfast," bringing us closer to our fun-loving and pajama-clad neighbors and friends. Last I checked, we're in the throes of an obesity epidemic threatening our children with shorter lives than ours for the first time in a century. Still, the pleasure principle seems to trump all logic.

Here's the problem, or part of it: health professionals are prejudiced in favor of knowledge. We paid tens or even hundreds of thousands of dollars for our education and have spent our lives gathering and refining knowledge about diseases. So we think information can solve any problem. Typical is Harvard cardiologist Peter Libby's in-the-box assessment in his medical journal commentary on the unfinished business of cardiovascular risk reduction: "Despite meaningful progress in the identification of risk factors and the development of highly effective clinical tools, deaths from cardiovascular disease continue to increase worldwide. . . . Although lifestyle modifications, such as improved diet and increased exercise levels, benefit general health and the metabolic syndrome and insulin resistance in particular, most people continue to resist changes in their daily routines. *Thus, physicians must continue to educate their patients regarding an optimal balance of drug therapy and personal behavior*"(Libby 2005; emphasis mine).

I'm a bit of a public health geek, so you know I'm all for knowledge as a general principle. But knowledge alone is neither necessary nor sufficient to produce behavioral change. I want to scream when I hear my colleagues say, "If only they *knew* how the way they eat is contributing to their diabetes . . . heart disease" . . . you pick the disease. And I want to scream even louder when I read public health articles that show how much people learned from a particular program but don't even mention whether this new knowledge helped them live healthier. Usually it didn't. The general public is ahead of the health profession on this—two-thirds in a recent poll did not believe that lack of knowledge was related to obesity in society (Fuemmeler et al. 2007).

The answer, and what I'm advocating in this book, is systems change to structure short bouts of group physical activity into our social interactions and cultural expectations, as well as our built environment. And we'd better get up to speed quickly to include it in the way we market active living. When we finally got past just telling adults to quit smoking and teens not to start, we made some real headway in tobacco control. When we built in some systems to keep people from drinking and driving, the death toll dropped dramatically. So now, when it comes to the obesity epidemic, we really have to stop expecting folks to swim upstream and resist not only their biological urges but also the well-financed and well-crafted seduction of the automobile, oil, highway construction, and entertainment industries. It's time to put the policies, regulations, and practices in place that will make it seem like people are swimming downstream, that will make it a lot easier for them to make the active choice and increasingly difficult for them to make the sedentary one. *Easier*, like getting the whole stadium up and dancing with the celebs during pregame or halftime shows at spectator sports events. *Easier*, like creating brief dance routines that people can do with their co-workers on company time. And *harder* to be inactive, like reserving nearby parking spots for the disabled, so that able-bodied workers, students, or shoppers have to do a bit of walking.

There are a few points of light. The growing "active living" movement shifts the emphasis from exercising for a set period each day to changing one's lifestyle to include activity throughout the day, like raking rather than blowing leaves, parking a little farther from our destination, and strolling with the dogs after dinner. Active living also focuses on making these kinds of activity easier by changing the built environment: well-maintained sidewalks everywhere, more and better recreational facilities, and walkways and bike paths connecting one part of a city to another. But active living is still dominated by strategies that require ongoing self-initiated individual action to engage in regular physical activity. Many neighborhoods have perfectly good sidewalks and parks but are rarely crowded. The reality is that walking paths and bike trails, exercise facilities, and fitness equipment are used consistently by the small segment of the population that is already relatively healthy.

Furthermore, it's hard to imagine working-class or poor neighborhoods, where it requires an act of God just to get potholes fixed and street lights replaced, being first in line for urban redesign projects. In reality, the lion's share of mixed-use development goes to affluent communities.

WHY A BOOK?

If we want to see the twenty-first century that the government's public health experts have envisioned for the nation and memorialized each decade in the US Department of Health and Human Services' Healthy People physical activity objectives, we need a catalyst, something similar to the aerobics craze of the 1970s, which began as a military-based study (more on this later) and spawned television shows and videotapes— not to mention a booming market for leg warmers previously coveted only by professional dancers. But the example of aerobics only goes so far. Regardless of media depictions, only a small percentage of people started doing aerobics. It wasn't a mass movement, and a mass movement is exactly what's needed right now. The purpose of this book is to make a compelling argument for a paradigm shift in our society's approach to physical activity promotion. At this juncture, as we face twin epidemics of obesity and sedentariness, we need a spark to propel our interventions from an incremental science-driven seepage housed in the public sector, into a surging advocacy-driven flood commandeered by—are you sitting down?—the private sector.

My focus is squarely on physical activity as the foundation or cornerstone of our ability as a society to reverse the accelerating erosion of our physical fitness and wellness. I believe that too much attention is currently directed toward eating and way too little is focused on activity. But, just as this is the first time in human history that we don't have to expend a lot of energy to consume food, so physical activity, by itself, will no more solve the problem than nutrition alone. This tension between a comprehensive wellness approach and an emphasis on physical activity will undoubtedly be apparent as the book unfolds. And that's perhaps as it should be, since it'll take a chorus of voices added to mine to figure it all out. After twenty years in public health, watching big failures and small successes, I'm just trying to change the tune and get us all on beat.

Let me tell you where I got my inspiration. In 1996, when I was making the transition from academia to the public sector, directing the health department of Richmond, Virginia, I spent a lot of time imagining how I could improve the fitness of an entire city. I knew I wanted to bring the department into the twenty-first century by focusing on chronic disease prevention and particularly physical activity promotion. But my challenge was to figure out how to inspire or induce people to do something that humans have tried to avoid throughout most of our history on the planet and that is still shunned in most forms by all but an elite sliver of the population. Sitting at my desk one day, I started thinking about the times in life when being active was strictly "fun and games," when it was play, not work. And since for me, especially during life transitions, daydreaming often inspires me to write a poem, out popped "Recapturing Recess."

Remember when we were kids? We could eat all we wanted—or all our parents could afford—and run all day without feeling tired. We could go from zero to sixty without stretching and warming up or hurting ourselves. We didn't have a dozen deadlines, a house to clean, parents to care for, and kids—and grandkids—to pick up after. Movement wasn't "exercise." It was joyous and *fun*.

Fast-forward to my arrival back in LA to start a chronic-disease division at the county health department. I thought, why not "recess" for adults? Recess breaks at work could boost energy levels, get the blood flowing back from the buns to the brain, alleviate stress, lift spirits—just as they do for kids! They could be done right in the work space, anytime, in any attire, by anybody. (After all, how many women dance the night away in tight skirts and on heels so high they'd break *my* ankles?!) It's "Instant Recess"! Just add music and shake your booty.

An *Instant Recess* break is a brief, low-impact, simple structured group physical activity for adults and kids. It's usually done to music and is integrated into the organizational routine at work, school, meetings, churches, sports stadiums, and other settings in which people gather. If we do it right, this relatively inexpensive approach could lay the founda-

---

Recapturing Recess

Now I know	And if you can recapture
Y'all can remember	Even a little of the joy
The recess bell	Of unbridled movement
The wave of exhilaration	Then just maybe
The sigh of relief	There's hope
The sheer release	For the *couch potatoes*
The transformation	Those of you
Of fidgeting	Too worn down
Into linear motion	Even to fidget
Raise up your hands	Think you need rest and food
If you can remember	But you toss and turn in bed
All that pent-up energy	And meals don't really sit well
Exploding	These bodies just weren't meant
Into air and space	For so much sittin' and standin'
And wind and sunshine	And so little *recess*

T___ ˙ *(April 3, 1996)*

---

tion for longer-term strategies. Granted, it won't solve all of our problems—it's going to take more than 10 minutes a day to completely arrest the epidemic of chronic disease and obesity, but it's a way of getting the ball rolling . . . a small *step* in the right direction.

Recess breaks make sense to most people and may be translated into action across many settings and sectors. It's a "push" strategy, which restructures the environment to make the healthy choices easy and the unhealthy choices difficult, the way smoking and soda bans push the antismoking and pro-nutrition causes. Call it a *sitting* ban! Other examples of "pushing" to make the active choice easier and the inactive choice harder include hosting walking meetings; supporting mass transit access with subsidized passes; restricting nearby parking and elevator use; and establishing automobile-free zones around shopping areas and employee drop-off locations. These strategies push, or nudge, people toward a socially desirable behavior, rather than pulling or beckoning them along, driven and sustained only by their own internal motivation. But both organizational *practice* and *policy* changes must be targeted, since practices implemented without policies in place don't have the institutional backing they need, and policies can be on the books without being implemented if there's no support among the people charged with getting things done. This will take top-down leadership and bottom-up grassroots support.

WHY THIS IDEA?

I think I come up with practical ideas and solutions to public health problems because I mostly "get it"—personally, not just professionally. I've lived a lot of lives in a lot of worlds during my five decades on the planet.

I grew up in Kansas City, Kansas—can't get much more middle of the road. I have since lived in most parts of the country, including the three largest metropolitan areas in the US—Chicago, New York, and Los Angeles. My father was an autoworker and World War II veteran who grew up on a farm in rural Louisa County, Virginia, and my mom was a second-generation teacher. Their marriage was working class meets middle class. My parents came of age during the Great Depression, and our current economic recession is what they always prepared me for. Like most lower-middle-class black folks, our family wasn't too far removed from belt tightening—both of them were from large families and talked about having to do without and go without . . . about using home remedies and being scolded for getting into any rough or risky sports because they couldn't afford a doctor. And our middle-class status was tenuous. We were a layoff or illness away from real struggle, which when I was growing up was a part of the daily reality of many of our relatives, neighbors, church members, co-workers, students, and classmates.

A child of desegregation, I learned early on to move comfortably in both white and black America, and to be fluent in standard English and in the colloquial "black English" dialectical vestige of slavery. I've been a poet since before I was or thought of being anything else. Being a writer helped me cope with the obstacles of isolation and discrimination I faced as I ventured out from my close-knit village of a black neighborhood, with plumbers and postal workers on our block, doctors and a state senator (Alex Haley's brother, George) on the next. I had to confront and navigate the perils of being the only African American or only girl, or both, in most every situation outside of church, family, neighborhood, and social gatherings—chess tourneys, German Club field trips, excursions with classmates to exotic (that is, Chinese or Mexican) restaurants, and Medical Explorer activities. I went to segregated public elementary schools, desegregated public secondary schools, elite small private institutions for undergrad and doctoral degrees, and a large public university for a master's degree. It took me fifteen years after getting my MD to pay off my student loans.

I was the last kid picked for sandlot softball games, and my first basket as a sixth grader in organized city league basketball was in the opponents' goal. (That was back in the day when only two of the six girls on each team were allowed to run the entire court—I didn't get that I was only supposed to play defense!) As I walked down the gauntlet of teachers and administrators "greeting" us on my first day of junior high, the only words spoken were the boys' basketball coach's exclamation that he wished I was a boy. We didn't have a girls' basketball team at school until my senior year of high school. But I inhaled sports, especially the Olympics. I played D-1 ball before they started giving women scholarships or letting women into the NCAA, so we toured the Midwest in station wagons and stayed in motels. I was a great shot blocker and a decent rebounder before those stats were tracked, but as an offensive player I had small hands that balls tended to bounce off.

I was a better basketball player at forty than I was at nineteen, when I gave up college ball to fit in biochem and molecular bio labs. But then basketball became something more than an enjoyable pastime. It became an essential part of how I restored my emotional equilibrium following difficult times during my first real "in your face" experiences of Southern racism, as the only black woman in my medical school class. That outlet's continued to serve me well over the years, particularly during the two-and-a-half-year battle for my appointment to a tenured associate professorship at UCLA, at the time one of only two underrepresented minority faculty with a primary appointment in public health . . . No great surprise for an institution that refused to tenure a serious scholar like Angela Davis, but I still never expected to become the *first* black full professor of public health in 2007, more than forty years after *Brown v. Board of Education.*

During five years of modeling and doctoring in New York, I was sometimes taken for Puerto Rican or Dominican, and many if not most of my patients were poor and Latino and recent immigrants. In an examining room, I'm about as likely to say, "Ponga su ropas" and "Respire profundo" as "You may get dressed" and "Breathe deep."

I was married for six years during medical school and residency. Sometime along the way after that, I figured out I was gay. Since we've gotten together, Darlene, my partner of nearly a decade, returned to school and finished community college and her bachelor's degree and is in grad school—definitely a dream deferred and now fulfilled for a teen mother from Compton who single-handedly put her daughter through Vassar undergrad and a University of Chicago master's program. Thanks to her, I now have a granddaughter—a little Blaxican, according to our Mexican American son-in-law, though I was never a mother. Which is probably just as well, because I feel like all these diverse experiences put me in exactly the right place, at exactly the right time, doing exactly what I was put here to do.

WHY THIS BOOK?

Many researchers have written public health books focusing on nutrition and arguing for large-scale approaches to obesity prevention and control that make healthy eating easier and eating nutrient-poor foods harder. Marion Nestle's *Food Politics* is a prime example. However, hunger, an innate biological drive, presents a different set of opportunities to intervene in promoting healthy eating compared with those available in promoting physical activity—*and* a different set of challenges. People have to eat, and they will generally eat healthy stuff if it's in front of them and the other stuff isn't. But there's no inherent urge for adults to hit the parks and sidewalks. More often than not, adults even manage to squelch kids' natural impulses to move, wearing the youngsters down to well-behaved mannequins.

Meanwhile, there's little incentive for the private sector to do the right thing. Encouraging people to eat nutrient-rich foods at the expense of processed foods is a losing proposition for the food industry. "Big Food" would lose money, because the profit margins are much smaller for nutrient-dense whole foods like fruits, veggies, and whole grains than for highly processed "faux foods" like sodas and fries. But the sports and fitness industry's interests *are* served by public health efforts to increase opportunities for physical activity. These companies will make more money if efforts to get the population moving succeed. So there should be less push-back from the private sector in getting people active than in getting them to eat healthy.

There are also many books that summarize scholarly work on physical activity and health from an environmental standpoint. However, these books focus on the physical or built environment. Their discussions of the social, political, and organizational environments influencing physical activity are rudimentary at best and essentially tone deaf on cultural influences. Nor do they devote much space to sorting out the levers for change on a broad scale. Oil, auto, tire, and road-construction industry lobbyists will not stand idly by and allow public infrastructure funds to be redirected from highways and suburban streets to mass transit systems and pedestrian-friendly urban centers.

Last, but not least, this book breaks down some silos between public health folks from different fields and backgrounds, especially nutrition and exercise. Probably because I had hard-science training *and* practical experience in hardscrabble public health clinics and foster care agencies before going into public health research, I tune in to biological, physiological, and psychological interactions on the "runway" (the individual level), and social and organizational interactions at "18,000 feet" (the community level). For example, physical activity has long been known to mitigate weight gain beyond just the modest number of calories burned while active. I highlight the indirect effect of modest-intensity activity in lifting mood and decreasing the overeating often associated with stress and depression. I also point to the direct effect of exercise in increasing cognitive processing efficiency. Enhanced cognitive or executive functioning may facilitate our ability to defer the immediate gratification from eating fatty, sugary, and salty foods and pursue loftier goals like improving our fitness and health (Kessler 2009).

INSTANT RECESS . . . IN A NUTSHELL

What's needed now is a popular approach to mobilize leadership and galvanize change. To build the momentum needed to improve fitness on a large scale, we need modest changes in physical activity through low-intensity intervention across America. Then we can move to the radical restructuring of the physical, social, and cultural environments needed to permanently and consistently support active lifestyles. But we constantly have to contend with the lack of sustainability of investments in individually targeted education and counseling programs, and this will continue to plague us until lawmakers and regulators revamp the infrastructure. Unfortunately, we have neither the political will nor the operational know-how at this point to get that done.

In the meantime, we can focus public health leaders on small steps we can take *right now* to increase physical activity, to start the ball rolling. In *Instant Recess*, I argue that the only viable solution in the short-term is to reacquaint people with small amounts of movement through organizational "push" policies and practices designed to make being active the default choice. The "pushers" in this case are institutional leaders, like pastors and bosses, whom public health advocates must convince that instituting regular recess breaks will not only improve their congregants' and employees' health, but also increase productivity. In the case of corporations, that translates into profits. In the case of religious institutions, that translates into members who have more energy to do good work and earn more with which to tithe. Not coincidentally, this top-down approach also eliminates the need for individual volition to initiate change.

In this book, I offer a way to bridge the chasm between the public health community and the rest of society. I appeal to leaders everywhere to look in the mirror and accept responsibility for the health of their charges. The *Instant Recess* approach should be able to reach almost all of the public whose health we want to improve, and tap into common cause among government, corporate, association, foundation, religious, and nonprofit institutions as employers and beneficiaries of the human capital upon which they rely.

In the following chapters, I'll outline a sophisticated but straightforward and digestible analysis of the problem of physical inactivity in American society. I'll provide backup from study findings, many from my own research team, that illuminate the sociocultural influences on physical activity. In particular, I'll be talking about *solutions*—levers that might be used immediately to promote and disseminate constructive change.

The time is ripe to create a groundswell of support for making physical activity an essential ingredient of daily life—for our own personal and our collective good. In their book *Nudge*, the behavioral economists Richard Thaler and Cass Sunstein (2008) argue that public policies should be designed to take human nature into account, thereby making it "easier for people to choose what's best for themselves, their families, and their society." Creating environments that make the healthy choice the easy choice is not new to public health. It was memorialized by the World Health Organization's Ottawa Charter, the first-ever international conference on health promotion, in 1986. Fortunately, some folks outside public health are beginning to get on board with this perspective. Obviously, recess breaks have become my favorite vehicle for "nudging" our society toward a healthier, more active way of structuring our lives. By the time you finish this book, I hope you'll understand why.

ONE The High Price of a Sedentary America and the Challenge of Getting Society Moving

THE LURE OF THE COUCH IS
COSTING US AND KILLING US!

Health

Unless trends change quickly, the current generation will be the first to lead shorter and sicker lives than their parents (Olshansky et al. 2005). Many of them won't live to see their grandchildren!

Hollywood images aside, being sedentary is the norm in America. According to the National Health and Nutrition Survey, 95 percent of Americans do not get enough physical activity (Troiano et al. 2008), but even that figure is an underestimate of Americans' love affair with their couches. We get an average of 10 minutes of moderate to vigorous physical activity every day, at best, and spend most of our waking time—

more than nine hours per day—sitting, reclining, or lying down (Owen, Bauman, and Brown 2009).

That's the national average. Physical activity levels are even lower in less affluent or ethnic minority populations. In Los Angeles County, one of the most culturally diverse locales in the nation, more than 40 percent of residents report *less* than 10 minutes of continuous physical activity per week (Yancey, Wold, et al. 2004).

Physical inactivity drives up the risks for many chronic diseases (Physical Activity Guidelines Advisory Committee 2008; Breslow and Breslow 1993; Mokdad et al. 2004). It's on a par with smoking and high blood lipid levels as an independent risk factor for heart disease and stroke, and it also increases the risk of diabetes, osteoporosis and hip fractures, breast and colon cancer, Alzheimer's disease, depression, and other chronic conditions (Physical Activity Guidelines Advisory Comm. 2008).

Physical inactivity also contributes to the energy imbalance producing obesity.* Obesity is pandemic in modern society, with two in three US adults now classified as overweight or obese (Ogden et al. 2006). Obesity and sedentariness are a lethal combination driving illness, disability, and death. Obesity not only exacerbates inactivity-related health conditions but also adds a litany of indirectly related problems: cancers of the uterus, ovary, prostate, esophagus, stomach, lung, pancreas, rectum, and liver; gall bladder disease; knee osteoarthritis and gout; low back pain; increased risk from anesthesia; reproductive hormone abnormalities, impaired fertility, and fetal defects; and sleep apnea (US Department of Health and Human Services 2001). The epidemics of obesity and sedentariness are projected to take a tremendous toll on American health, productivity, and economic growth, exacerbated by the browning and graying of the population. Sedentariness and obesity are clearly eroding

*Overweight, in adults, is defined as a body mass index (BMI) of 25–29.9 kg/m^2 (the weight in kilograms divided by the square of the height in meters, or about 703 times the weight in pounds divided by the square of the height in inches). Obesity is defined as a BMI of 30 or more. Morbid obesity is defined as a BMI of 40 or more. The definitions differ in children because of their growth patterns. Overweight is defined as being between the 85th and 95th percentiles of a growth chart derived from children's height and weight data from the 1960s to 1980s, and obesity is defined as being at or above the 95th percentile.

the strides we've made in fighting heart disease and diabetes (Olshansky et al. 2005).

I spoke of the browning of society: lower-income communities and communities of color continue to be plagued by higher levels of obesity and illness, disability, and death due to chronic diseases (Flegal et al. 2002; Truong and Sturm 2005). For example, among middle-aged Americans, 60 percent of white women were overweight or obese in 2001–2, compared with 80 percent of black and Mexican American women (Flegal et al. 2002).

Childhood obesity is a growing problem (Ogden et al. 2006; Freedman et al. 2006). About 16 percent of school-age children and adolescents are obese (Ogden et al. 2006). That's a threefold increase in young kids, and a fourfold increase for teenagers, from past decades. In communities of color, childhood obesity is much more common (Freedman et al. 2006). Rates of overweight and obesity top 50 percent in many urban school districts (Slusser et al. 2005). A similar escalation in excess weight has even occurred in infants and toddlers (Wang and Lobstein 2006).

Wealth

The dangerous combination of expanding waistlines and pervasive sedentary behavior may spell disaster for the health, economic, and social security of the United States. Beyond the high toll on individuals and families from loss of earnings, job and income security, and retirement flexibility, the costs are mounting for employers. Physically inactive or obese workers have higher rates of absenteeism, attrition, health care costs, injury, short- and long-term leaves, and workers' comp claims (Anderson et al. 2005; Chenoweth 2005). Moreover, from the standpoint of the company's bottom line, productivity and morale are down and "presenteeism" (occupying your chair but doing little or no work) is up among these employees.

At a time when youth are increasingly at risk for diabetes and heart disease, health care demand and costs for young workers are expected to rise considerably over the next few decades. This will coincide with the time of peak demand from aging baby boomers, overwhelming

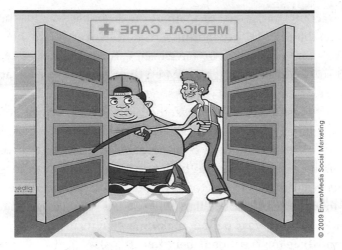

Figure 2.   During the next decade, baby boomers will increasingly have to compete with Gen Xers and Yers for health care.

our medical care system, and the nation's increasing ethnic diversity— over half ethnic minority by 2060 (Yancey, Bastani, and Glenn 2007). However, the intangible costs of obesity are also highly significant: fewer years of productivity and a diminished quality of life, like not living to see your grandchildren grow up. Medicare data suggest that obese seventy-year-olds will spend 40 percent more time disabled than normal-weight people of that age (Lakdawalla, Bhattacharya, and Goldman 2004). Personal losses due to the obesity crisis are not as easy to quantify but do have a tremendous impact on society. These costs will only escalate as obesity continues to affect younger and younger populations.

Sedentariness and obesity affect not only our national productivity but also US corporations' global competitiveness in a tightening economy. Physical inactivity has become so commonplace that the costs imposed on society by people with sedentary lifestyles (for example, for the treatment of diabetes and other chronic diseases in the uninsured) rival those imposed by smokers and heavy drinkers (Keeler et al. 1989; Sturm 2002). In fact, the majority of the population fails to achieve the amount of regular activity necessary to maintain a desirable weight—no matter how little they eat! US expenditures related to overweight, obesity, and low levels of physical activity have been estimated at 27 percent of the total costs of health care in 2005. More than 10 percent were attributed to physical inactivity alone (Anderson et al. 2005).

Obesity is estimated to have cost the United States $117 billion in 2000 and $147 billion in 2008 (Finkelstein et al. 2009). In California alone, the total direct and indirect costs of physical inactivity, obesity, and overweight were more than $21 billion in 2005 (Chenoweth 2005). That's $638 per resident, $1,516 per worker, and $28,011 per work site—or one out of thirteen health care dollars. These costs were projected to rise 32 percent over a five-year period, making a convincing case for effective and immediate intervention (Chenoweth 2005).

Meanwhile, resources are short and dwindling. A survey distributed to the health officers from seventeen of the largest US metropolitan areas revealed that on average less than 2 percent of their budgets were allocated to chronic disease even though chronic diseases account for 70 percent of all deaths nationwide (Georgeson et al. 2005). Another startling stat from the Centers for Disease Control and Prevention is that public health measures like enforcing housing standards and ensuring clean water were responsible for twenty-five of the thirty years of life expectancy added during the twentieth century. But the lion's share of the $1.3 trillion spent annually on health went to curative medicine, which added only five years to our lives (Kessel, Beato, and Royall 2004). And if chronic disease overall gets little funding, physical activity's share is minuscule. My colleagues and I reported in a review published a few years ago that few schools of public health or local health departments have physical activity programs (Yancey et al. 2007). The California Department of Public Health, for example, the largest state health department in the nation, only recently increased the number of employees available to address the physical activity needs of more than 33 million residents, from two to thirteen (Dorfman and Yancey 2009). Consequently, attention to physical activity has often been assigned by default to nutrition staff with few additional resources and variable levels of interest or training in the subject.

THE CHALLENGE: THE DECK IS STACKED AGAINST US!

The American Nightmare

It may sound odd after all those dismal figures, but Americans are highly motivated to get fit. Starting or resuming exercise regimens is the most popular New Year's resolution, mostly because of our desire to lose weight. Obesity is almost universally stigmatized in mainstream American culture, particularly in women. Being heavy is equated with stupidity and laziness. One study found that the quality of life for a severely obese child is equivalent to that of a pediatric cancer patient undergoing chemotherapy (Schwimmer, Burwinkle, and Varni 2003). And being skinny is equated with intellect, drive, and attractiveness. Americans spend $40 billion a year on weight loss products (Bryant 2001). At any given time, more than one-third of men and nearly half of women say they are trying to lose weight (Timperio et al. 2000). But only 5 percent, at best, of people who start weight loss programs achieve long-term success (Mann et al. 2007). Most people only exacerbate the problem by repeatedly losing fat *and* muscle, then regaining only fat. This amplifies the trends toward heavier and less fit Americans seen since the 1970s. This is, in large part, an unintended consequence of the generally greater focus on dieting for quick results on the scale, with insufficient attention to, or success at, increasing physical activity, particularly resistance exercise.

So what exactly is the solution to our collective yo-yo attempts at fitness, leanness, and wellness? Better understanding the problem is the first step toward solving it.

Biology Is Destiny

Genetically, we haven't changed much from our hunter-gatherer and agrarian ancestors. We have been programmed by evolution over the millennia as behavioral opportunists—to avoid exercise as adults and to prefer sweet, salty, and fatty foods (Eaton et al. 2002; Rowland et al. 2008). These predilections enhanced our survival odds during famine. For most of our history on this planet, we expended more than 5,000 calories every day securing food and shelter and escaping or elimi-nating predators (Bellisari 2008). There's no intrinsic biological drive concomitant to hunger that prompts activity in adulthood. Quite the contrary—conserving energy for utilitarian purposes probably kept our ancestors from starving. Acquiring enough calories for survival at the lowest possible energy cost has been a powerful selective force through-out human evolutionary history (Bellisari 2008; Katzmarzyk and Mason 2009; Landsberg 2008; Reaven 1999). So people who disdained activ-ity in their leisure time probably had a survival advantage, and most of us got those genes! But that was thousands of years ago. Why are we fatter and less fit than our mothers and fathers? Little change has occurred in leisure time physical activity during the past several decades of the accelerating obesity and chronic disease epidemic, suggesting a significant decrease in obligatory or incidental physical activity as the culprit (Brownson, Boehmer, and Luke 2005). Obligatory activity, unlike exercise per se, is utilitarian in nature, not aimed at enhancing health or enjoying leisure time. Certainly, even as dietary quality erodes, calorie density and portion sizes—along with the ever-growing palatability, accessibility, and commercial marketing of food—are expanding right along with our waistlines and contributing to "diabesity" (Kaufman 2005; Passe, Horn, and Murray 2000).

Movement Squeezed Out of Work, Leisure, and Transport

Americans didn't suddenly lose our discipline and resolve—times have changed! We're surrounded by a plethora of people-moving machines and seductive entertainment that keeps us riveted to our seats, just as we're inundated with a smorgasbord of succulent, pervasively and insidiously marketed, cheap, highly processed, nutrient-poor but calorie-dense foods.

Good ol' American ingenuity in engineering and technology develop-ment has robbed us of the need to burn calories as we move (more often sit) through the day. People used to be paid to be active because many jobs required hard physical labor. While there are still many low-wage jobs that are extremely demanding physically (such as hotel workers who clean ten to fifteen rooms an hour, or dockworkers who unload shipped goods), overall occupational activity has plunged, while sitting has skyrocketed. Labor-saving technology and globalization have shifted workers away from agricultural and manufacturing occupations and toward service and entertainment jobs, which demand far less energy. Computers, e-mail, text messaging, webcasting, and other technology-based communications continue the trend toward small but significant reductions in calorie burning across a broad range of types of work.

The other major trend, this one partially subsidized by the federal government and supported by commercial interests, is the increasing use of private transportation, favoring the car over the pedestrian, bicyclist, or transit rider. Walking or biking churns through calories, and even catching trains and buses requires more walking than driving door to door. So while leisure time activity has remained stagnant, the proportion of US workers commuting by car, truck, or van has increased over the past several decades, as has the use of autos for all types of trips (French, Story, and Jeffery 2001). Based on Department of Transportation data, calculations by the Centers for Disease Control and Prevention suggest that one in four trips we took in the late 1990s was less than a mile and that three in four of those were made by car (UCLA School of Public Health 2003). Kids commute, too—to school. Two-thirds walked or biked to school in 1974, but that dropped to less than 15 percent in 2001 (US Centers for Disease Control and Prevention 2007). That means millions of kids losing an excellent, easy opportunity to burn off some of the pop and chips they eat at lunch.

Urban sprawl and suburbanization have contributed to our dependence on automobiles. This is a result not only of limited or inconvenient public transportation and mega-malls but also of a lack of sidewalks, protected crosswalks and bridges, foot or bike paths connecting neighborhoods or areas of a city or town, and other pedestrian amenities. Public policy has also undermined active leisure. Tax dollars have gone to spectator sports like stadium construction rather than community recreational facilities. School physical education has traditionally been geared more toward cultivating elite athletic talent for revenue-generating collegiate and professional sports, such as men's football and basket-ball, than teaching kids skills for lifetime physical activity pursuits for their leisure time. This hurts the vast majority of youth, especially girls, as I discussed in a *Richmond Times Dispatch* editorial (1997), "Sports Are Good for Girls," when I was a local public health director. Athletics, I wrote,

> can decrease their engagement in risky behaviors such as substance use and sexual activity, prevent depression. . . . Importantly, developing athletic competence can help focus girls more on what their bodies can *do* than just how they *look*. Small triumphs in sports can support the confidence and self-esteem for independent and aggressive pursuits in other areas. . . .
>
> In our society, however, engagement in physical activity has been considered unfeminine. This parallels the far-too-frequent overshadow-ing of competence by appearance in its treatment of women.
>
> Women are told how to look, act and be, and are ridiculed or labeled derisively when they don't conform. That message is obviously received and validated by pubescent girls. For instance, middle school girls of color in focus group studies conducted at UCLA and the University of Texas identified an unwillingness to disturb their hair and make-up as the primary barrier to their participation in exercise. Not surprisingly, another major barrier was gender inequity in their instruction by male PE teachers. In the words of one girl, "[I]f there's only one ball, the boys get it!"

When you consider that 100 percent of kids need to establish the habit of activity for health and less than 1 percent will ever make it to college or pro sports, the selfishness and shortsightedness of this approach is criminal.

Television watching, still the leading offender in riveting us to our couches and chairs, is ubiquitous in the United States and, increasingly, throughout the world, and it contributes in several ways to obesity and chronic disease. It's an extremely appealing, mesmerizing, addictive, and completely stationary way to spend leisure time; its ads encour-age the consumption of high-fat, high-sugar foods; and people are par-ticularly likely to snack while watching TV. The magnitude of the effect varies, but more TV time consistently correlates with a higher prevalence of overweight and obesity and poorer dietary patterns. However, the association between screen time and physical activity is neither clear nor consistent. Teenage boys, for instance, watch more TV (especially sports) *and* engage in more sports and other active recreation than teenage girls or most any other demographic. Thus, televised sports and other physical activities may have redeeming value in launching people off the couches and onto playing fields and ball courts. My partner and I certainly hit the tennis courts more often during the slams.

People movers and labor savers have rendered most incidental or obligatory physical activity at home obsolete as well. Strenuous house and yard work involving walking, pushing, pulling, sweeping, scrubbing, wringing, hanging, raking, weeding, laundering, lifting, washing, and carrying is no longer absolutely necessary for survival. Even activities that we still do regularly demand less exertion. For example, backbreaking, calorie-incinerating snow shoveling is now done by modern snowblowers that barely require lifting a finger. Leaf blowers have replaced rakes in many garages. And cheap immigrant labor means that the middle class, not only the wealthy, can buy relief from such chores. In fact, some do-it-yourself physical activities are actually discouraged for reasons related to the public good— for example, using dishwashers and professional car washes conserves water and electricity.

The less people have to do, the more quickly they get tired when they exert themselves just a bit, which of course discourages them from exercising. Americans more and more readily opt out of any meaningful amount of movement. In fact, a Mayo Clinic study found that people who were overfed decreased their walking by one and a half miles per day, and that obese people walked three and a half fewer miles per day than lean ones (Levine et al. 2008). The majority of walking occurred in short bouts (less than 15 minutes) at low intensity (1 mile per hour).

Bombarded by Encouragement—in the Wrong Direction!

Commercial marketing exploits sedentary human tendencies. The food industry also disingenuously tries to deflect attention from its contribution to the obesity epidemic by supporting sham physical activity promotion. It's basically just PR—all spin, no substance, like buying a few jungle gyms or producing a few staid and boring public service announcements that nobody watches. Aside from undermining meaningful changes in food and nutrition systems, this drives a wedge between the already disjointed public health nutrition advocacy and exercise-science interests (discussed in greater detail later in this chapter). It may also fuel controversy that would discourage the fitness industry from investing in promoting physical activity to avoid being drawn into bad publicity on obesity issues.

Look beyond Big Food, and it's interesting that the businesses that make and sell the goods and services that compromise fitness are not even on the public health advocacy community's radar screen. These include highway construction contractors; oil, tire, and automobile manufacturers and retailers; television and film companies; suburban developers; video game and TV manufacturers and distributors; video and DVD rental companies; and spectator sports. Nor are we on their radar screens. Attendance at a 2005 Institute of Medicine invitation-only industry roundtable on childhood obesity shows how few inroads public health advocates have made in spotlighting the culpability of industries that promote sedentary behavior. None of these companies were represented, in stark contrast to the high profile of soda manufacturers and fast-food retailers who promoted their product reformulations (albeit still highly processed and nutrient poor) to cut calories, fat, and portion sizes. The only physical-activity-related companies in attendance were those promoting activity—physical video gaming and sporting goods.

Commercial inducements are especially problematic in underserved communities. So here's an all-too common conundrum facing parents: A huge new McDonald's just opened at a busy intersection in Compton, a city in southern Los Angeles with many very dangerous neighborhoods. The restaurant features an expansive kids' playground—shiny, clean, attractive, and fenced in. And of course the restaurant hires round-the-clock security guards. If you're a parent, where do you take your kid? Or send them when you're juggling jobs? The nasty neighborhood park where they could get harassed by gangbangers, pricked by a needle, or shot in a drive-by? Or McDonald's?

My research team at UCLA worked with investigators from several other universities across the country to examine how outdoor advertising contributes to obesity-related health inequities (Yancey et al. 2009). We found that schools and day care centers in low-income or predominantly ethnic minority zip codes have many more ads for sugary drinks and fast food in their immediate vicinity than those in wealthier or whiter zip codes. That's not so surprising, but we also found that ads for TV shows, films, video games, and cars were much more pervasive in these communities. And ads promoting physical activity are nearly nonexistent in any area—we found only 38 of them among 2,233 ads, or less than a percent, across six cities. However, in high-income white zip codes, which had only 4 percent of total advertising sheet space, 36 percent of the ads were for physical activity. It goes without saying that ads for gyms, sports, and fitness equipment nearly always featured relatively young muscular men and thin women in affluent-appearing surroundings, not "people like us." And advertising in these areas in general was pretty sparse—there were so few ads in affluent white communities in the Los Angeles area that we had difficulty finding a zip code for inclusion. We chose Pacific Palisades, near the ocean between Santa Monica and Malibu, as a last resort. The only ads there, other than realty posters on bus benches, were concentrated along the main commercial corridor and clearly aimed at workers rather than locals. This wasn't hard to discern, since they were mostly in Spanish, and very few Pacific Palisades residents are Spanish-speaking Latinos!

School Complicity in Cooping Up Kids

The role of K–12 schools in student inactivity is becoming more and more apparent (Trost 2004). There are PE requirements in forty-eight states, but they're rarely enforced or sufficiently funded because of cutbacks in funding for PE and the diversion of students' time to reading and math by No Child Left Behind. The issue is not only quantity but quality. It won't help to mandate additional physical education minutes if those minutes translate to more time wasted sitting or standing around. In less affluent schools, overcrowded classes, inadequate staffing, broken water fountains and restrooms, and "temporary" classroom trailers encroaching on playground space strewn with cigarette butts and crack vials don't exactly encourage kids to move and sweat during recess and physical education.

My research team also conducted a study of public school PE and related policies, programs, practices, and participation in California (UCLA Center to Eliminate Health Disparities and Samuels & Associates 2007). Our findings underscore the uphill battle. We demonstrated that students were moderately or vigorously active for only 5 to 7 minutes of a typical 30-minute PE class in most schools in less affluent areas. Both lower fitness test scores (conducted annually on all California fifth, seventh, and ninth graders) and lower standardized test scores were linked to lower levels of moderate to vigorous physical activity during PE class. Also, few elementary schools had full-time PE specialists on staff, and many had none. Most elementary school playgrounds, and PE classes at all levels, were overcrowded and underequipped. Schools, on average, fell far short of the ten-day, 200-minute (elementary) or 400-minute (secondary) PE-participation requirement. So kids whose neighborhoods are rundown and unsafe, and whose parents are working two jobs and commuting long distances, without the time to drive them to soccer practices or the money to pay city recreation program fees, are literally stranded. Their chances of getting a meaningful amount of daily activity outside school are slim to none.

Cultural Conspiracies against Active Living

America's growing diversity will drive even greater public investment in treating "sedentary behavior disorder," because obstacles to physical activity are greater for certain segments of the population. Combinations like being older and female, or poor and of color, can be especially daunting. In many low-income single-parent or two-wage-earner families, discretionary time is far from leisurely—sucked up by long work hours or household responsibilities for child care or elder care. Kids aren't often sent out to play in low-income areas because of parental concerns that outdoor activity is not safe, especially for girls. Media attention (such as Amber Alerts) stoke parents' fear of "stranger danger" even in more affluent areas. Especially in tough economic times, blue-collar frustration manifests more often in good ol' boy gatherings in front of flat screens to watch sports than getting out on courts and fields and playing them. Age comes into play on the opposite end of the spectrum when seniors or even their younger relatives, fearing injury, are reluctant to join a walking club or exercise class. Or they simply subscribe to the attitude that seniors deserve a rest. And socialization that equates sports and exercise with masculinity is common among immigrant and first-generation Latinos and Asians. That may be great for guys' health, if not their maturity, but it reinforces the notion that the female sex is physically fragile and easily injured. Girls and women from these communities are among the least active Americans.

ETHNICITY

The history of certain groups in this country, such as African Americans and Latinos, may also influence attitudes toward physical activity. Having experienced generations of forced manual labor, material deprivation, and discrimination necessitating walking inordinately long distances while others rode in cars and on school buses, and limited opportunities for higher education and white-collar jobs, people from these ethnic backgrounds tend to view physical exertion negatively, even if generations removed from these struggles. This may explain a study by my mentor and colleague Shiriki Kumanyika, who found that older African Americans were skeptical of their need for activity outside of work, citing the need for rest at the end of a long day . . . despite the sedentary nature of most work now. The intentional avoidance or low prioritization of physical activity makes sense in this context. And people who have been quite sedentary, especially those who are overweight, tire more quickly—even by such ordinary activity as climbing a flight of steps. This translates into profuse sweating, aching joints, and heavy breathing on a short walk that would require little effort for a fit person, which is discouraging and may reinforce negative cultural attitudes.

Ethnic differences in TV watching may also contribute to lower physical activity levels among African Americans, American Indians, and other groups. Data from a California statewide survey on teens' TV habits found that about 50 percent of white male and 60 percent of white female adolescents watched two hours or less of TV per day, not a huge amount, relatively speaking (Babey et al. 2005). But only a third of their African American peers reported this modest level of TV consumption. Safety concerns also contribute to high levels of TV watching among children living in low-income urban communities. Parents' well-grounded fears of violence often compound more common concerns about traffic injury, making them reluctant to allow their children to play outside. More times than I can count, I've heard parents say that they'd "rather have a fat kid than a dead kid," and I don't blame them. Parental fears about sexual assault may lead to even greater restrictions for girls.

Increased TV exposure may be particularly detrimental for adolescents of color. A media content analysis revealed more than four times as many noticeably overweight "black prime time" actors as those on general-audience prime time (Tirodkar and Jain 2003). This compares with less than a twofold black-white difference in obesity. Though I can't prove it, ethnic differences in the value of being thin may influence the decisions of advertisers and casting agents, distorting television reality. These culturally targeted media depictions may reinforce ethnic obesity stereotypes (Aunt Jemima) and create the impression that obesity is normative and even embraced in the black community. This distortion may also reinforce class- and ethnicity-based norms of excess weight, which may then color body-image ideals and the pursuit of these ideals. In other words, if you're a teenage black girl, and your mom, aunts, and older sisters are all overweight and inactive, and you watch a lot of TV and many of the actors you see are overweight, sitting a lot and gaining weight may seem inevitable. The handful of active black women on TV are serious athletes, and that's not you!

And that brings us to the hair factor. Yes, the hair factor. Women in some ethnic groups can't quickly restore their 'do after a full sweat, so they're not going to muss it without a compelling reason, not when many a Saturday is spent at the beauty shop, and each trip costs not only hours but also half a paycheck to achieve conventional straight hairstyles. Chris Rock's 2009 film, *Good Hair*, is no joke. Hair's an issue for all women, especially with the mainstream cultural ideal of straight, blonde hair screaming from every TV commercial and billboard. But if

Blue Grease

When I was about five,
I thought that hair grease
Would magically transform
My fine, limp, frizzy, nappy, kinky,
     short
Cross between my mother's and
     father's,
Fuzzy-edged, broken-off kitchened,
Crop screamin' homage to my
     African ancestors
Into the long, flowing, head-
     shaking, Breck-shining,
Northern European vintage locks
Of the white girls and women on
     TV.

So one day
I stashed that big, ol' jar o' Posner's
Into my schoolbag
An' after kindergarten
After gramma dozed off
I slathered that stuff on my head
'Til time got better.

My ribbons from my carefully
     coiffed
Mother-crafted three-braided 'do
Of that morning

Were saturated and blue-hued with
     Posner's.
And I still had the same
Fuzzy-edged, kinky-kitchened,
No-flow hair.

When my mom picked me up
She inquired
More calmly than I'm sure she felt
About the change in my hair.
I feigned ignorance.
She cooperated in the charade
And dropped the subject.

Years later
When I recalled the incident
I realized that my mother
Never applied adjectives like "good"
     and "bad"
To hair
And always referred to summertime
     outdoors
Tanning my already carmel skin
As getting "brown as a berry."
Maybe that's why
This is a poem
And not The Bluest Eye.

                    T___' (April 10, 1995)

you didn't grow up in the black community, I think it'd be hard to grasp the extent to which its daily "care and feeding" rule girls' and women's lives. Maybe you can get a glimpse from my poem, "Blue Grease."

GENDER

Women, in general, are more sedentary than men, and the lowest levels of physical activity are reported among ethnic minority girls and women because of the many obstacles they confront. An interesting difference between men and women highlighted above concerns whether or not people think they're overweight. Our UCLA–Los Angeles County Department of Public Health team recently studied survey data from a diverse group of non-obese individuals (normal weight or less than about 30 pounds overweight). The most striking finding was that women were much more likely to think that they were overweight than men . . . not surprising, given the socially imposed pressure most women feel to fit into whatever body type men find attractive (Yancey, Simon et al, 2006).

"Action follows thought," as a friend says. Out of all the groups we studied, all men and Latinas and African American women were *less* active if they perceived themselves to be overweight. Most people think that heavier people are less active, but our data suggest that it's *thinking* you're heavy that's linked to less activity, not *being* heavier, at least for the two-thirds of us who are not (yet) obese. (Similar findings associating inactivity with self-perceived overweight, rather than actual overweight, have been reported in children.) White women were the only ones surveyed who were *not* less active if they thought they were overweight. That's fortunate in one respect, since many more white women think they're overweight than do women of color or men. But they weren't any *more* active if they perceived themselves to be overweight either.

Of course, for obese folks, it's a different story. Obese women, for example, reach more than half of their peak aerobic capacity (how much work their heart and lungs can do) after only 2 to 4 minutes, even at a snail's pace—the 2½ miles per hour rate identified as "comfortable" by most women in that weight-status category (Ekkekakis, Lind, and Vazou 2009).

So public health messages trying to convince people that they're overweight to get them to exercise are most likely misdirected. Our data show that almost all obese people already know they're overweight (Yancey, Simon et al, 2006).

Most of us tend to do better when we feel better, not worse, about ourselves. And excess fat carries a huge stigma, apparently even if it's only in our minds. In fact, once a marker of prosperity, fat suddenly became a scourge at the end of the nineteenth century, and this social disapproval has only increased since that time (Kersh and Morone 2002). I've always found it interesting that the socially desirable weight status for women is typically associated with affluence. When food was hard to come by, Rubenesque figures ruled. As technology and politics made food cheap, especially low-quality and highly processed food, thin women—alternating between waiflike, and toned and fit—have graced the society pages and fashion-magazine spreads. But it is quite apparent that this scrutiny of weight and preference for thinness is imposed primarily on women: much heavier (and older and less glamorous) men than women regularly gain admittance to the ranks of the "beautiful people."

I know the *weight* and pervasiveness of social norms to look skeletal because of my own personal experience of pressure to conform to a particular body type. When I went from a segregated elementary school to a desegregated junior high—basically that meant being among a few black students in a sea of whites—I suddenly felt totally oversized. Of course, pushing 6 feet at age eleven, that wasn't entirely surprising. But at 130–135 pounds, I'd *never* before felt fat—never even thought about it! Around the white girls obsessed with thinness who were my constant companions at school, I began to diet and, as a budding scientist, to experiment with diets. I remember weighing myself and calculating my caloric input with great precision at the height of the grapefruit craze, in an effort to determine whether it really burned fat. Fortunately, my mom, ever the pragmatist, assured me when she saw that I was substituting celery and carrots for lunch on weekends, that I was not overweight, didn't even have the genes to be overweight, and should be eating those foods as a between-meal snack. Luckily, I listened. But the stigma of not adhering to mainstream norms heaped upon those already negatively stereotyped can be particularly detrimental. Consequently, black women and Latinas typically dismiss messages that smack of such portrayals (like obese, lazy, and stupid welfare mothers).

Some say ramping up the stigma is just what's needed. Political science professors Rogan Kersh and James Morone (ibid.) include demonizing the user as one of the seven necessary steps of government intervention in examining the politics of obesity.

However, this viewpoint distracts us from a focus on the behaviors that need to be changed, namely, more activity. The "demon user" in other social movements refers to the consumer of a product or service, or person engaging in a behavior, not a personal attribute like weight. Our society glorifies sedentary behavior in film and video game ads, in the status conferred on certain cars, and the subtle derision aimed at people who are diligent exercisers as "gym rats" or "exercise freaks." Conversely, we have yet to aggressively promote routine activity in ordinary individuals, as opposed to gifted athletes in revenue sports. If stigmatizing obesity hasn't worked in ninety-five years, it seems unlikely to do so now.

Berkeley, California–based media-studies experts Lori Dorfman and Larry Wallack (2007) echo this concern, in that the obesity framing moves the conversation "downstream," to a focus on the individual rather than the social and physical environmental conditions that foster or inhibit physical activity for the whole population. This is a bonanza for commercial interests, as Big Food blames people for their gluttony, laziness, or lack of discipline, and self-serving Big Pharma medicalizes the problem and points to drugs and surgery as the solutions.

Meanwhile, in contrast to boys and men, girls and women typically lack encouragement, facilities, and role models for leisure time athletics. These biases affect even highly accomplished women. About fifteen years ago, I was on a panel with another physician, an internist and mother of two in private practice who lived in an affluent black area of Los Angeles. She approached me after the session, in which I'd made the point about hurting girls this way, acknowledging that she, too, was culpable. She didn't blink at spending $100 or more on a pair of sneakers for her son, but balked at spending that much on athletic shoes for her daughter.

What girls and women *are* encouraged to do is package themselves in whatever style of dress they've been socialized to find attractive. Women routinely sacrifice comfort and ease of movement for the aesthetics of close-fitting dresses and high-heeled shoes. I suspect that figures into my observation, whenever I'm in Atlanta at the CDC for a meeting, that the scientists and managers take advantage of the lovely art-decorated, music-piped-in, and carpeted stairwells, but the sistas, mostly administrative support staff in stiletto pumps and tight skirts, are congregated at the elevators. This goes along with traditional views of femininity that discourage sweating and aggressive play because it's not ladylike. At the extreme end of the spectrum, some Latina grandmothers in one of our study focus groups expressed concern about a possible loss of virginity from certain types of vigorous physical activity, that horseback riding, gymnastics, or martial arts would rupture girls' hymens, thereby shaming their families and diminishing their marital prospects.

It's really not surprising that my internist colleague was predisposed to associate athletics with her son but not her daughter. I recently ran across an article in the August 5, 1954, issue of *Jet* magazine (target audience: working- and middle-class African Americans) titled "The Truth about Women Athletes." I had a good idea of what the article was about, but I was still appalled to actually encounter it in print. The whole gist seemed to be to reassure the audience that pro baseball player Toni Stone, boxer Gloria Thompson, and tennis star Althea Gibson were not lesbians and switched from being the "hard-bitten, sexless and sensational" athletes they were in the ring or on the court or field to the "kind of women that make men turn their heads." This, despite the fact that the pinnacle of athletic achievement is often captured in images of African American women. It reminded me of my freshman year in college, when Woody Hayes, then the venerable Ohio State football coach, claimed that all women basketball players were lesbians—apparently a fate worse than death! And the beat goes on. We've progressed as a society, but I still hear teen girls' concerns that weight training will make them "muscle bound" like body builders. And I was truly outraged by conservative talk radio host Don Imus's on-air riff a few years ago disparaging the Rutgers women's basketball team as "rough" "nappy-headed 'hos" that could readily be confused for (male) NBA players. Worse yet, I didn't see a single black woman commentator or athlete of any stripe, as best I could tell, among the pundits fueling the media blitz in the immediate aftermath, as the denigrating comments were relentlessly replayed.

Even ads for gyms and sporting equipment primarily target men, while women—especially older women, women of color, and women already carrying some extra weight—tend to feel quite uncomfortable in most commercial gyms. An exploratory research study we conducted in the late '90s at UCLA was aimed at improving fitness and reducing cancer risk among African American women through nutrition education and gym-based exercise at a black-owned facility. We evaluated the relative success of different recruitment strategies. Women with less formal education and those who were already overweight were more likely than thinner women to enroll through word-of-mouth contact, apparently needing personal reassurance that the study was for people like them. We convened focus groups to probe the participants' responses to the program. They communicated their discomfort with other exercise environments when surrounded, in their words, by "skinny white women." As I mentioned earlier, however, even skinny white women are not immune to self-defeating attitudes. Studies show they're not exercising for health but aiming for a level of thinness that few can achieve, especially after age 30. In other words, they feel they have to look skinny to look good, and white men are more likely than men of color to agree, adding to the pressure and self-loathing with which many continually grapple, which not infrequently devolve into eating disorders, especially in adolescents.

An earlier study of high school students found that white girls had highest rates of vigorous physical activity among all girls (28 percent), with lower rates among Mexican American girls (21 percent) and African American girls (17 percent) ("Vigorous Physical Activity among High School Students—United States, 1990," 1992). The passage of Title IX, the 1972 legislation barring sex discrimination in public education, has greatly expanded opportunities for girls and young women in sports. In 1972, only 3 percent of girls were involved in high school sports nationwide. That exploded to nearly one-third involved in 2002 (Weiner 2004). Title IX changed society's views of girls and women as athletes. In fact, ever since the 1996 Olympics in Atlanta, I can barely get my 6-foot-2-inch frame through an airport without someone asking me what WNBA or college team I play for. I was never approached as an athlete when I actually played Division 1 college basketball thirty-some years ago—when shorts were really short and post players weren't confused for football linemen. (I'm number 25 taking the jumper in the old school photo.)

I still remember the exhilaration of that time around the '96 Olympics: Sheryl Swoopes on the cover of the *New York Times Magazine*, staring down

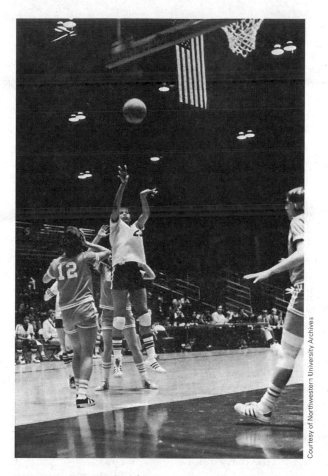

Figure 3. At Northwestern University, the author hits
the outside jumper (circa 1977).

the camera with a basketball in her hand like a serious playa! The launch
of not one, but two women's professional basketball leagues—first, the
American Basketball League (ABL) the fall after the Olympics, where the
serious but non-superstar athletes played, and then the Women's NBA
(WNBA) the following summer. The commercially appealing superstars
defected to the WNBA after the NBA suddenly realized that there was
a market for women's professional basketball. The NBA put the ABL out
of business a couple of seasons later by threatening corporate sponsors,

We, Too, Are Ballas

She rose this week
To the rim
Above the rim
Made a highlight film
Threw it down
Hung on the rim
Chinned up and kicked out
Landed with a Shaq-style grimace
Got T'ed up
Didn' matta
'Cause she took us up with her
On her broad back
On her lithe legs
On her strong shoulders
Made us PROUD
LOOOOUD and rowdy
In our living rooms
In sports bars
At college and pro games
Made me rise a little higher
To throw his shot into the bleachers
The only sensational play
These 43-year-old knees
Can still parlay

And when we hit the playgrounds
School gyms
Driveway hoops
Any court
With a cylinder

Poised to accept offerings
Of our hopes and dreams
Of equality
Equity
A level playing field
Title IX indeed
Not just in name
And plans
And schemes
And memories
Of cheers
And glory
And adulation
And promise

Sheer joy
Of bodies in motion
Of striving, thriving and deriving
The last ounce
Of energy, determination
Frustration at any limitation
Engendering
Fearlessness
In other arenas
In which ovaries
Give us
Competitive advantages
Over cojones!

T___ *(January 29, 2001)*

like Sears and State Farm Insurance, with a boycott if they continued to support its competitor. I'd written a lot of poetry about male athletes, but had always wanted to write a poem about women's basketball. When I saw Michelle Snow cap off a fast break with a two-handed dunk a few years later for the first time in organized competition, I had my inspiration for "We, Too, Are Ballas."

INCOME AND RESIDENCE

The risk of physical inactivity and the burden of inactivity-related conditions and diseases fall disproportionately on poor and rural communities, and on residents of the southern United States. Despite the "walkability" of many inner-city neighborhoods in terms of narrow streets, short blocks, and mixed land use, the environments in these communities are less conducive to activity than average. And the average is already pretty unfriendly. Few pedestrian amenities such as sidewalks and traffic-calming devices like speed humps; heavy traffic but few people walking outdoors; uneven terrain, few private or community gardens and little park space; poorly maintained recreational facilities when they exist at all; locked-up school playgrounds; aesthetically unappealing surroundings; gang presence and a feeling of danger (whether or not police statistics bear this out)—all conspire to keep people in these communities rooted to their chairs and couches. Psychologically, noise, traffic congestion, information overload (pervasive ads), overcrowding, and neighborhood disorder also increase stress and strain and constrain activity participation. This is compounded by the time and money crunch stressing many poor and working-class families, in terms of arranging for child and elder care, working long hours for low pay and little if any paid leave, having no flex time or say in how to get the work done, and commuting long distances because of the lack of centrally located, affordable, and desirable housing in most large metropolitan areas.

Back to Title IX. A Harvard study showed that African American and Hispanic high school girls participate in sports at about half the rates of boys, while white girls' rates were comparable to boys': 54 percent and 58 percent, respectively (National Women's Law Center and Harvard School of Public Health 2004). A 2007 Harris Poll found that urban girls enter sports at an older age and participate less than boys, while gender parity has essentially been achieved for suburban girls and boys. Moreover, 55 percent of urban girls (read: poor or working-class, black or Latino) describe themselves as nonathletic, more than twice the proportion of boys (26 percent), and only 9 percent of girls are highly athletically involved, less than half the proportion of boys (19 percent).

Same ol' story. These urban girls, in cities across the country, have been called the "left-behinds of the youth sports movement" (Thomas 2009). Girls are forced to shoulder more household and child care responsibilities than boys, particularly in immigrant families with more traditional gender roles. For Latina girls and women, for example, few Olympians and even fewer professional athletes of their ethnicity are in the media limelight. Instead, they get *Ugly Betty*. Girls' and women's sports are not highly valued by American society in the way that boys' and men's are. That translates into inequitable investment by schools and communities in the development of male and female athletes, even if only tacitly in the unfair way that private resources (financial support, volunteer time) are distributed to fill gaps in low-income districts and neighborhoods. That also translates into families not viewing girls' sports participation as a path to upward mobility in the way that they often do boys' participation. Maybe they should consult Richard Williams, Venus and Serena's dad!

THE SCIENCE-INDUSTRIAL COMPLEX

Combine our "hard-wired" genetics with our obesogenic environment, and it's easy to see how small caloric excesses and energy deficits produce "weight creep" over time. A mere 1-pound-a-year weight gain means that normal twenty-year-olds will become obese fifty-year-olds. Just as they reach their peak periods of productivity and leadership, the chronic conditions accompanying their obesity—diabetes, high blood pressure, heart disease, stroke, arthritis, depression, cancer, liver disease, and many others—will steal their energy and undermine their well-being, performance, and functioning.

But quiet as it's kept, and odd as it seems, we don't have proven treatments to help people achieve and sustain substantial weight loss (Mann et al. 2007), despite the billions of dollars spent by the pharmaceutical industry to convince us otherwise. We've invested more than 40 years of intervening at the individual level in research samples of affluent volunteers, without substantive, sustainable, or widespread effect. The four decades of scientific research focused on the individual have also failed to provide the guidance to get and keep most people active. As I pointed out earlier, trying to educate or counsel people into active lifestyles just hasn't worked, and our perseverating, tic-like, in this individual approach as a professional and scientific community is mind boggling. After all, one definition of insanity is doing the same thing over and over again and expecting different results. For example, motivational interviewing (a personalized counseling technique) added to an environmental change intervention in black churches produced a clear additive benefit for fruit and veggie intake, but not for physical activity (Resnicow et al. 2005).

Science is built on and sustained by incrementalism—infinitesimal contributions that don't stray far from mainstream thinking and generally maintain the status quo. Senior investigators populate federal and foundation grant-review committees and journal editorial boards, the gatekeepers of the flow of scientific evidence. Nearly all of these investigators come from affluent backgrounds and hail from disciplines focused on individual lifestyle-change counseling, clinical treatment or rehab, or the unique needs of elite athletes—psychology, medicine, physical therapy, and exercise physiology. The halls of the academy are mired in sameness, and there are powerful vested interests in maintaining the status quo. It's not exactly fertile soil for game-changing solutions.

Culture Counts!

This raises the specter of another challenge to our coming up with novel policies, practices, and programs that work in the real world to increase physical activity. The public health bureaucracy is dominated by older, affluent white men and their cultural perspectives (representation of women is still spotty at best at the highest levels). Not having professionals in leadership positions who reflect the growing diversity of America is hurting our health and fitness as a nation.

Health campaigns for such costly epidemics as obesity, HIV/AIDS, and substance abuse have often failed, in no small measure, because Eurocentric leaders don't recognize and account for culture. Because the term *culture* has become almost a cliché, let me pause here and share a favorite quotation on the subject. Some might find it simplistic, but I think that if more health professionals and government leaders embraced this sentiment, they might be a little less self-righteous and presumptuous about their own objectivity. The writer W. Somerset Maugham (1943, 16) captured it eloquently:

> It is very difficult to know people and I don't think one can really know any but one's own countrymen. For men and women are not only themselves, they are also the region in which they were born, the city, apartment or the farm on which they learned to walk; the games they played as children; the old wives' tales they overheard; the food they ate; the schools they attended; the sports they followed; the poets they read; and the god they believed in. It is all these things that have made them what they are and these are things you can't come to know by hearsay. You can only know them if you have lived them. You can only know them if you ARE them.

I think of this quote when I hear some pediatricians lament—often with an air of superiority—that Mexicans just can't seem to understand that they're overfeeding their babies. Many recent Latino immigrants come from places where diarrhea is the number one threat to infant health. To them, babies who are not plump are at risk of dying from the cold and flu viruses that all babies get repeatedly! When health professionals fail to acknowledge such cultural notions, proclamations like "Your baby's too fat!" ring hollow. Besides educating the mother, in a noncondescending manner, about the lesser risk of diarrhea and other wasting diseases here, a culturally proficient recommendation might recognize the collectivist and family-focused nature of most Latino enclaves. Such a recommendation might encourage parents to play active games with their kids to promote healthy brain development, to set a good example of being active for their kids to follow, and to advocate for more physical activity during the school day to help their kids concentrate better and learn more in school.

I've also frequently run across the Marie Antoinette "If they don't have bread, let 'em eat cake" mindset. A colleague at a federal advisory committee meeting scolded me for suggesting that promoting personal responsibility was not a useful public health approach to obesity prevention and control. He bragged that all he did was cut out chips and walk a few times a week, and he dropped 20 pounds in six months. I asked if he lived in a pricey neighborhood or on a main drag with cars speeding by at 50 mph, whether he had a health club membership or access only to a gang-infested park, whether he generally ate out at upscale restaurants or picked his meal off the dollar menu or from the food truck vendor. I don't think I swayed him, since his perspective on people without those luxuries is that they're not smart or hard-working enough to improve their station in life. But it's imperative that we acknowledge and do more to assure conditions in which people have healthy and readily accessible alternatives, and that those alternatives are the expected ones, the default choices. As my colleague Bill McCarthy likes to say, "Freedom of choice is truly illusory in many communities." In a society growing more diverse by the moment, it is more important than ever that we start building a bigger tent (in terms of age, socioeconomic status, race, ethnicity, and acculturation) to sharpen our cultural lens and broaden our competencies.

It's puzzling that so many public health professionals are convinced that knowledge is the missing element in getting people to change their behavior. Nutritionists have about the same obesity rates as others of similar education and income, and they know a lot more about what they should be eating. We all know that we should floss and brush several times a day, but most of us rarely do so. I often ask for a show of hands, when lecturing at professional conferences, of how many people used the gym or hit the sidewalks during the past twenty-four hours of being ensconced in a nice hotel in an invariably nice neighborhood. It's unusual when more than one-third of my well-educated, often well-heeled colleagues respond affirmatively. Or, alternatively, I ask everyone to stand and then run through a laundry list of health behaviors, requesting that audience members sit down if they don't regularly adhere to the recommendations. Needless to say, I've never exhausted my list with anyone still standing, including me! If the 30 minutes of daily physical activity doesn't get them, the sleeping seven to eight hours a night or flossing after every meal does. What we do routinely is affected much more by

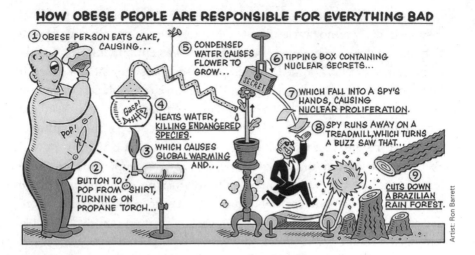

Figure 4. Our obsession with thinness instead of fitness deflects attention from the physical inactivity we should be stigmatizing.

how we feel about it, how we weight it during the hourly trade-offs necessary to maintain our overscheduled lives, and how others we care about or spend time with feel and do than it is by what we know about it. We'd better learn how to hit 'em where they feel, not just where they think!

Sometimes the messenger's as critical as the message, and messages indicting fat folks are usually coming from skinny Minnies. I have to watch out for this myself. Though I'm far from what I consider thin (that was my modeling weight of 140–145 pounds, not my usual 35 pounds heavier now), people see me as genetically endowed for leanness and athleticism. Would that that were the case, and I didn't have to fend off the spare tire like everyone else, less and less successfully, I might add. But things are as they seem. So I have to work harder to make sure my obesity-control advocacy isn't interpreted as an indictment on obese people. A colleague of mine, Oscar Streeter, who's carrying a bit extra in the middle, is much more direct, making it a "we" and not "you." He challenges his patients to get moving by grabbing his love handles and making fun of his recently diagnosed pre-diabetic condition. "I've got it and I've got no choice but to deal with it, but it's a daily, sometimes moment-by-moment struggle!" Besides, while weight is a vital health indicator, there's no need to focus on weight in a public health campaign. If the focus is put on food and activity, the weight will take care of itself over time—time measured in generations unless we turn the tide soon.

This emphasis on the behavior, not the girth, also addresses recent concerns (including mine) that the prevention component of federal health care reform focuses outside the clinical setting, especially on the workplace, and that employee wellness incentives follow ethical guidelines (Goetzel 2009; Pearson and Lieber 2009). Effort should be rewarded, and people should be held responsible for their behavior, not their biometric indicators like weight that are governed by genetic endowment, life circumstances, and many other factors beyond the control of the individual.

Moving the Needle

"Upstream approaches" are strategies that operate at a broad societal or even global level and influence the behavior of whole population segments at once. For example, legislation or regulations that redirect tax dollars to mass transit from highway construction would get a lot more folks moving than establishing walking programs at churches. But walking programs would reach more people than physicians prescribing exercise for their patients. All of these approaches are useful, but scarce resources have to be prioritized to get the biggest bang for our buck. Approaches that address social norms, popular culture and organizational values, financial incentives and disincentives, and our physical surroundings are beginning to succeed in other arenas where the old models of individually directed education and behavioral management have failed. This is true across the board and is not a radical notion. Some of our greatest public health successes came about only after public health officials acknowledged the importance of culture and societal norms, particularly in influencing children and youth.

Early environmental tobacco-control advocates did not wait for the science. They were of the "Damn the torpedoes!" mindset: do something first and study what you've done later. Like-minded colleagues who've spent time in the practice as well as in the study of public health express this so well. "If you want more evidence-based practice, you need more practice-based evidence," says Larry Green at the University of California at San Francisco. Ross Brownson at Washington University in St. Louis likes to quote Immanuel Kant: "It is often necessary to make a decision on the basis of information sufficient for action but insufficient to satisfy the intellect." And one of this country's pioneers in cancer control advocacy, my friend and mentor Helene Brown, has always asserted poignantly that we'd be successful in spite of, rather than because of, academia.

Previous and unsuccessful tobacco-control intervention approaches, developed by psychologists and physicians, were in keeping with the current physical activity promotion paradigm. These approaches focused on persuading adults to quit smoking because it was bad for their health, and getting kids in schools not to start smoking for the same reason. They took the form of smoking-cessation admonitions in clinical settings and smoking discouragement as a part of health education curricula in schools. Conclusive evidence that smoking bans decreased smoke exposure, despite their considerable "face validity" or intuitive appeal, was years away when such bans were already widely imposed.

Similar evidence is mounting for the link between physical inactivity and poor health. But, unlike physical activity—a necessary (albeit diminishing) part of daily life, tobacco is a nonessential, addictive substance. Furthermore, most smokers got addicted when they were minors and, in theory, legally barred from purchasing or using tobacco. This opened legal avenues for interrupting access. In addition, smoking affected nonusers by subjecting them to secondhand smoke. The harm and discomfort to nonsmokers caused by this involuntary exposure was strategically leveraged in enlisting public support and outrage.

Such conditions as direct harm to others, especially youth, haven't been met to the same degree for sedentary lifestyles as for tobacco. The ultimate societal impact of exposure to a sedentary lifestyle, however, may be comparable to the now-well-documented toll of tobacco use. Also unlike tobacco, we don't yet have any clinical tests to accurately measure physical activity participation or relate that "dose" to chronic-disease risk. It's kind of hard to scientifically prove the physiological effects of too few neighborhood role models for physical activity or too many for being plastered to a chair. Nor are policy solutions as politically or logistically straightforward. Intervening to actively engage the majority in a protective behavior in a democratic and individualistic society is considerably more complex than intervening to passively prohibit a health-compromising behavior embraced by a small and declining minority.

Thus, environmental strategies to promote physical activity, while a burgeoning area of interest to policy makers and legislators, are still in an early phase of development. The 2009 reauthorization of the State Children's Health Insurance Program, or SCHIP, included funding for a demonstration project that will work toward the construction of a comprehensive, systemic model for the prevention of childhood obesity (Oberlander and Lyons 2009). Individual-level intervention alone—one-to-one or group nutrition counseling or exercise instruction, for example—has been the centerpiece of most efforts to control chronic disease, and its limitations are increasingly apparent. Unfortunately, environmental change approaches have yet to permeate health policy in a way that is likely to engage the majority of Americans in regular activity.

TWO The Benefits of Widespread Physical Activity and Opportunities to Move the Needle

THERE'S ALMOST NOTHING EXERCISE CAN'T FIX —
OR AT LEAST IMPROVE ON A BIT

Health

If exercise came in pill form, it would turn up in every medicine cabinet in America and make some Big Pharma companies very wealthy indeed. As a matter of fact, one goal of industry-funded research is to discover oral medications that mimic the effects of exercise training, so-called exercise mimetics that can combat metabolic disorders—so far to no avail (Hawley and Holloszy 2009). Physical activity is one of the most potent and grossly underutilized tools in preventive medicine's black bag. Getting as little as 50 minutes of moderate to vigorous physical activity per week confers some health benefits; getting 150 minutes or more weekly is associated with a full spectrum of protection across most health domains (Physical Activity Guidelines Advisory Committee 2008). Physical activity lowers your chances of getting heart disease, high blood pressure, diabetes, stroke, breast and colon cancer, osteoporosis, Alzheimer's disease, depression, and anxiety disorders. Activity may even decrease the length of the first stage of labor (Lawrence et al. 2009).

Physical activity also prevents weight gain and is often singled out as the key to keeping off lost pounds. This may be one of its most critical roles in health, as most of the chronic diseases mentioned above are also linked to obesity. Because of its positive influence on body weight and body composition, activity indirectly protects against a number of other chronic conditions, including gall bladder disease, fatty liver, many cancers, sleep apnea, infertility, fetal defects, low-back pain, and gout.

Modest amounts of physical activity may actually offset the increased medical costs and other adverse consequences of overweight and obesity (Hu et al. 2003; Stefan et al. 2008; Pescatello and VanHeest 2000; Wang et al. 2004). Physical fitness, the bodily manifestation of adequate doses of physical activity, protects against death from many causes, including heart disease, stroke, metabolic disorders (Blair et al. 1995; Haapanen-Niemi et al. 2000), and nonalcoholic fatty liver disease, independent of weight (Church et al. 2006). Studies have demonstrated that obese individuals who are fit have much lower death rates than normal-weight individuals who are unfit (Physical Activity Guidelines Advisory Committee 2008), but that's a bit misleading, since most people lose weight while becoming fit. Some even argue that fitness entirely erases the risks of fatness (Katz 2009), but that's a minority view. Physical activity also helps to treat and manage many chronic diseases, such as diabetes, osteoarthritis, and depression. Exercise is a regular part of rehab from breast cancer and heart attacks, and it is increasingly seen as an important adjunct to the recovery and restoration of functioning after a variety of insults.

Beyond disease prevention and control, physical activity promotes optimal functioning and well-being, increasing attentiveness and the efficiency of cognitive processing. It improves sleep quality (King et al. 1997; de Jong et al. 2006), regulates mood, lowers heart rate, improves energy, enhances sexual enjoyment, serves as an appetite suppressant, and burns abdominal fat preferentially (that is, it burns proportionately more abdominal fat than fat on the extremities) (Physical Activity Guidelines Advisory Committee 2008). It decreases our taste for highly sweetened beverages and increases our preference for water and water-bearing foods like fruits and veggies (Passe, Horn, and Murray 2000; Sturm 2008; Westerterp-Plantenga et al. 1997). After all, after you've been working out and sweating—and hopefully that's been recently enough for you to remember—you probably don't want a soda.

How physical activity exerts its protective influence varies by disease. For example, activity is known to increase HDL ("good") cholesterol, decrease triglycerides, and improve heart muscle efficiency (militating against heart disease and stroke); to consume calories needed for tumor growth, improve immune system functioning, postpone pubertal development, and regulate reproductive hormone levels (helping to prevent cancer); and to decrease gastrointestinal transit time (helping to prevent cancer and diverticulitis).

Given the widespread sedentariness of Americans, there is considerable opportunity for even small increases in average activity levels to have a large positive population impact. Diabetes risk has been shown to be 50 percent lower among individuals physically active *at any level*, and 66 percent lower among those at least moderately active (James et al. 1998). It's been estimated that if the physical activity levels of the entire US population increased by 30 minutes of brisk walking each day, coronary heart disease risk in women would decrease by 30 to 40 percent and colon cancer incidence would decrease by 15 percent (Colditz 1999; Wolin et al. 2009).

In terms of cumulative benefit—whether activity broken up into short bouts delivers the same return as longer intervals—the influence on health seems to be similar (Physical Activity Guidelines Advisory Committee 2008). In the Harvard Nurses' Health Study, for example, investigators found that merely avoiding sedentary behaviors (like TV watching) as well as engaging in light activities such as ironing or washing dishes protected women against developing diabetes and obesity over the six-year period of observation (Hu et al. 2003). More recently a group of investigators found that 3-minute bouts of physical activity ten times per day lowered serum triglycerides to the same extent as one continuous 30-minute bout of physical activity (Miyashita, Burns, and Stensel 2006). However, longer bouts are likely necessary to achieve and sustain high levels of aerobic fitness—that is, heart and lung capacity and efficiency (Physical Activity Guidelines Advisory Committee 2008).

There's a lot of discussion swirling around right now about how much additional activity would be required across the population to arrest the epidemic of obesity. Most estimates range from 3 to 10 minutes per day. Longer periods, in excess of 30 minutes per day, have also been put forward. However, those longer estimates that I've run across seem to be based on European populations that are much healthier than Americans. For example, my colleagues Michael Costanza and Alfredo Morabia (Costanza, Beer-Borst, and Morabia 2007) produced an estimate of about 45 minutes per day, based on Swedish adults—16 percent obese, about half the rate in America, and much more active. (Swedes have higher rates of active transportation such as biking and riding mass transit, higher requirements for physical education and sports in schools, and a greater adherence to those requirements, presumably leading to better-habituated and better-conditioned adults.) It takes less activity to make a sizable dent in fitness or fatness in a heavier, more sedentary, and less fit population.

Wealth

From the standpoint of costs, being regularly active even at middle age and older is linked to substantially lower health care expenditures. One study found 5 percent lower costs for health plan members active for at least 30 minutes just one day a week (Pronk et al. 1999). In a more recent study, these costs—including medical, pharmacy, X-rays, lab, co-pays, and deductibles—were $3,453 for everyday exercisers, $3,594 for those active five or six days a week, $4,442 for people exercising one to four days a week, and $5,684 for the sedentary. That's about 3 percent higher costs for every day without exercise (Bland et al. 2009). Physical activity may also offset the adverse health consequences of mild obesity. This adds up to a lot of potential benefit to employers. One study found a $250 savings in health care costs for physically active versus sedentary employees overall, and $450 in savings among active versus sedentary obese workers (Wang et al. 2004). Research has also shown that every dollar invested in work-site health promotion yields $3.50 to $6.00 in savings from reduced absenteeism, increased productivity, and lower health care costs, and an average 30 percent reduction in workers' comp and disability claims costs (Aldana 2001). Most importantly, when the environment supports individuals who are changing their behavior, 80 percent maintain that change for two or more years (National Diabetes Education Program 2007). These outcomes of work-site health promotion programs have to be interpreted in light of the considerable selection bias involved—healthier workers are more likely to enroll and continue in these programs than sedentary, overweight, or unfit ones. But that bias understates rather than overstates the likely advantages, since again, it takes less exercise to make a dent in a less healthy population.

At a societal level, a 10 percent decrease in physical *in*activity (people getting off their chairs and couches, but not necessarily making it to 30 minutes of exercise a day) is estimated to be able to reduce direct health care spending by $150 million annually (Colditz 1999). California alone might save more than $1 billion annually if the population of physically active and lean adults increased by just 5 percent (Chenoweth 2005). Of course, by decreasing or controlling obesity, physical activity may indirectly help to avert the costs enumerated in chapter 1.

THE OPPORTUNITY: A LITTLE GOES A LOOONG WAY

Where Do We Stand? Or Sit?

Societal paralysis and apathy are still the rule, although the climate is changing dramatically. This may be both a function and a reflection of the past decade of media attention to the escalation of the epidemics of sedentariness and obesity. The greatest traction in pursuing community solutions to these epidemics is in addressing childhood obesity. But focusing exclusively or even primarily on children's environments will *not* stem the rising tide. Going back to the smoking analogy, this point is exemplified in the success of a Port Arthur, Texas, tobacco-prevention initiative. The proponents' multilevel approach—spanning media, enforcement, cessation, and school and community involvement—was effective in decreasing smoking among youth *and* adults.

Just as small but widespread environmental changes created the obesity and chronic-disease epidemics, so, too, can small calorie-intake deficits and modest increases in exercise arrest excess weight gain and make Americans healthier. The gap between calories burned and consumed is small if you look across the entire population. Of course, that's not to say that there aren't much greater discrepancies at the individual level for dedicated couch potatoes downing mega-burgers and "grande" burritos, fries, pan pizzas, doughnuts, cupcakes, mocha lattes, and six-packs of soda or beer! Estimates suggest that the modest average energy imbalance could be offset by as little as an extra 5 minutes of moderate to vigorous physical activity a day. That equates to 10 additional minutes of exercise a day at work or school (for example, a brief structured group-activity break), assuming that at least half that time is of at least moderate intensity—the equivalent of a nondisabled adult walking at 3 to 4 miles an hour. Given that the average person now gets just 6 to 10 minutes of physical activity at that intensity level each day (Troiano et al. 2008), that little extra activity could go a long way. (It could be 50 percent or even 100 percent more than they're getting now.) And the societal benefit of arresting people's weight gain doesn't even take into account the chronic-disease protection that activity delivers apart from weight control. Nor its disruption of long periods of sitting, which some physiologists contend is just as detrimental to health as not getting at least 30 minutes a day of moderate-intensity activity.

The Built Environment

There's more and more evidence that the built environment influences physical activity and weight. Many studies show that adults walk and cycle more for transportation in communities where it's conducive to do so: where there's mixed land use, connected streets, short blocks, frequent intersections, light traffic, rail access, and a higher density than in sprawling suburbs. People in these "walkable" neighborhoods also weigh less. Adults and youth who live near appealing recreational facilities or scenic outdoor features such as trees, flowers, and grass, bodies of water, and pretty vistas are, not surprisingly, more active. Programs that increase pedestrian friendliness, like sidewalk construction and traffic calming, may increase children's active commuting. Still, most studies showing that the built environment can increase physical activity are cross-sectional, rather than longitudinal or experimental, meaning that self-selection cannot be ruled out as the reason for this link. In other words, people who are more active may choose to live in more activity-friendly areas, and—keeping in mind our concern for the epidemics' reach into poor communities—people who live in these walk- and bike-able communities may have the means to live wherever they choose. A Harvard study bears this out. Lee, Ewing, and Sesso (2009) found no longitudinal association between changes in exposure to urban sprawl for movers and physical activity. Male alums who moved from more sprawl to more dense areas became no more active, nor leaner.

Federal, state, and local governments, and foundations concerned with health, like the Robert Wood Johnson Foundation, are exploring active-living community redesign initiatives, with possible benefits beyond making people more active. Such efforts could also reduce traffic congestion, preserve open space, enhance the quality of life, and improve air quality. The most developed of the initiatives, Safe Routes to Schools, included $1 billion in the 2005 federal highway bill for distribution to states to facilitate bicycle and pedestrian commuting (Boarnet et al. 2005). The burgeoning collaboration of public health and urban planning holds much promise but, realistically, will mostly benefit affluent communities—at least in the foreseeable future.

The Social Environment

If the active-living movement is making small strides on the built environment, it has barely begun to address the social environment, despite

Snapshots

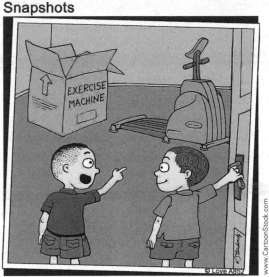

"Hey, we have one of those. You
hang your laundry on it."

Figure 5. Despite our best intentions, motivation
to lose weight or get healthy is rarely enough to
make most of us "roll solo."

the fact that social support, networks, and conformity pressures influence physical activity participation at least as much as—and I'd say more
than—the physical environment. Otherwise, how is it that groups living
literally side by side in the same neighborhoods can have such different physical activity levels? I've seen this time after time: the contrast,
for example, between relatively poor immigrants from Asia and those
from Latin America, the former congregating in whatever space is available—a park or a parking lot—early every morning to do tai chi, while
the latter have no such daily ritual. Most communities have a lot more
people who sneer at physical exertion than those who embrace it. Even
those who voice appreciation for active lifestyles acknowledge that they
don't often "walk the talk." But those same people may *actively* embrace
certain pastimes that are not specifically defined as exercise, like garden-
ing, sightseeing, and even shopping (but not on the Internet).

In part, the limitations of our current science reflect the difficulty in defining, measuring, and incorporating social and cultural environments in our activity-promotion research. Social norms, values, expectations, and roles are overarching elements of the environment that may mediate or modify the effects of the physical environment or may influence activity independently. The sociocultural environment hasn't been examined as closely as the physical environment, in part because of the interests and skill sets of the investigators traditionally working in this area. It's just now becoming an active area of investigation. However, as I suggested earlier, vestiges of our evolutionary programming or ancestral heritage may still leave most people equating any kind of real exertion to pulling teeth. Which explains why it often takes rehab from a heart attack or cancer treatment to lock in an active lifestyle, like the threat of our teeth falling out finally getting us to floss religiously.

If the active-living movement is a bit blind to the social environment, it's tone deaf on cultural norms and values—although these cultural assets are widely recognized outside academia, especially by corporate marketers. Specific cultural norms, values, and traditions that could facilitate physical activity, but are commonly underappreciated by researchers, include the dance tradition in African American and Latino communities, the encouragement to "be strong early in life" among American Indians, spiritual mind-body practices like martial arts among Asian Americans, and seniors' desire for social interaction and to maintain independence. Line dancing is extremely popular these days with adults and youth—the moves on Beyoncé's "Single Ladies" music video went viral in days. (Every black party I go to includes dancing that at some point morphs into the Cupid Shuffle or Electric Slide. Shades of the bus stop and the Village People's "YMCA" from my own "old school" days.) One of my colleagues commented, rolling his eyes a bit, that he just couldn't get parents of the girls in one of his physical activity research projects to attend scheduled meetings. However, at least three or four family members would show up for dance recitals featuring these girls. Doesn't sound like a problem to me—sounds like a solution! He's a quick study, so he soon recognized his participants'

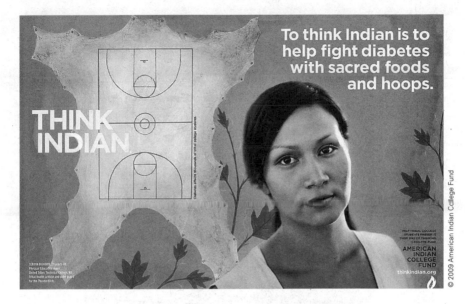

Figure 6. This "Think Indian" ad perfectly illustrates promoting health by means of embracing cultural values and traditions.

cultural appreciation of performance art as an asset and tacked on a discussion of the study before or after the recitals.

Adventures in Policy Advocacy

Many policy analysts say lessons from the campaign against Big Tobacco should inform anti-obesity efforts. One approach frames the battle against obesity primarily as public health versus Big Food, but there are pitfalls to this approach. The promotion of exercise by the food industry has created a backlash from public health nutrition advocates who say these efforts are intended to deflect attention from the industry's role in the epidemic and to deter policy solutions involving increased regulation or taxation. The food industry's promotion of physical activity focuses on changing individual behavior rather than on changing environments. Typical are philanthropic playground-equipment purchases and public education campaigns encouraging active recreation and

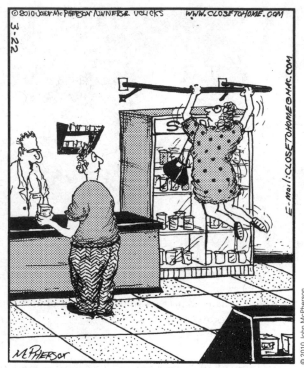

"Instead of passing the fat tax on soda, the government requires that people do 10 chin-ups before the cooler will open."

Figure 7.   On the surface, this is a tame and humorous nod to balancing our calories. From the standpoint of behavioral economics, however, physical activity is framed negatively, in this case as a disincentive to raising the price to deter soda intake.

admonishing families to take responsibility for their children's health. Fast-food companies have attempted to keep the focus on physical activity by highlighting snowboarding or beach volleyball in advertisements for hamburgers and fries. Their spokespeople do this by talking about "choice" and "balance." The emphasis on choice both absolves companies of responsibility for the accessibility of those choices and reinforces the inherently American belief that individuals are solely responsible for their own health, obfuscating the context in which the choices are made.

In other words, lobbyists could argue to lawmakers that Big Food is already helping fight the epidemic—of laziness. In an attempt to counter these claims that seek to hold Big Food harmless, nutrition advocates frequently make assertions like, "You'd have to run five miles to burn off that burger!" This framing implies consensus that exercise avoidance is strong motivation to deter overeating.

But demonizing the food industry as the cause of the obesity epidemic deflects attention from sedentary-behavior-promoting commercial concerns that have also contributed to the escalation of obesity, as earlier noted. Regardless of the industries targeted for exposé, aligning physical activity promotion too closely with obesity-control advocacy may be a liability. It risks the underappreciation of the full spectrum of benefits, ignores the fact that a desire to lose weight doesn't motivate people to take up physical activity in many culture groups, and could scare off fitness corporations who want to avoid controversy, adverse publicity, and guilt by association. By focusing exclusively on food-industry behavior, public health advocates may inadvertently collude with the "enemy" to exacerbate tensions between the fields of nutrition and physical activity. And I wouldn't put it past Big Food to have diabolically fueled this infighting.

At the same time, physical activity proponents, already a minority in public health circles and hungry for resources, have to resist being pimped by the food industry. These companies want to undersell their culpability and thereby avoid scrutiny and regulation or taxation by throwing pennies at school playground equipment and youth soccer programs while spending the big bucks to publicize these meager efforts. We should insist that food companies wanting to climb on board and be "part of the solution" do so by supporting large-scale environmental changes to increase physical activity participation population-wide. That will require substantial public funding, but these companies spent more than $23 million lobbying in 2008 (Center for Responsive Politics 2008). Public health nutrition advocates should reconsider their blanket criticism of the food industry if companies use their heft on Capitol Hill to support large-scale expansion of the public infrastructure for activity promotion such as bike lanes, parks, playgrounds, and public transit (Besser and Dannenberg 2005).

We should also adhere to some guidelines in accepting funding from industries that promote sedentary behavior *and* nutrient-poor food choices: for example, allowing only the logos for the health-promoting products such as Dasani or Aquafina and not Coke or Pepsi as a part of any public health social-marketing efforts (Dorfman and Yancey 2009; Yancey et al. 2009). Clearly, we should insist that companies genuinely interested in partnering with public health refrain from hitching their health-compromising brands to physical activity. In a later chapter I'll get back to this point in describing the attempts of the Professional Athletes Council and the San Diego Padres to grapple with these issues.

Organizing advocacy to promote physical activity is quite complex and goes beyond obesity prevention and control. It's not like substance control, where you can organize groups with similar and very clearly positive interests (health, safety) around preventing the use of a discretionary product, like tobacco or methamphetamine. But when it comes to advocating for exercise, the different interests may cancel each other out. Concessions to walkable-community design increase development costs. An investment in fitness staff and equipment channels money away from peer-support interventions. Putting more into PE at schools may be viewed as diverting money from academic goals, though a growing body of evidence suggests otherwise (see, for example, Trost 2004; 2007). People may prefer to spend their money on health and beauty treatments and other self-care services, which give immediate gratification, instead of spending time and money on health club memberships or lunchtime exercise. In other words, everybody sees their own resources as a finite pie, and they don't want a smaller piece for themselves. These perceptions are rampant, even if they're not grounded in reality. Focusing diverse interests on a unifying agenda to advance population physical activity has been difficult and slow to evolve. Because a large-scale expansion of opportunities, like adding a bike lane for every new car lane, will require substantial public funding, policy-advocacy efforts must be broad based. Public health departments and their constituents typically have limited experience in mounting or joining advocacy campaigns in arenas outside public health.

So we have to get smarter and identify as many leverage points as we can, even if it's outside our official area of expertise. For example, since there's so much potential traction in addressing issues affecting kids, we might focus on childhood obesity and highlight the growing evidence that physical activity and physical education improve test scores. The interests of environmental justice, asthma control, lead-poisoning prevention, and "green development" advocates converge with those of physical activity promotion in supporting neighborhood schools, mass transit, and tough air pollution standards. Another tool used to drive passage of aggressive school-nutrition policy in California was aggregating student-fitness data by state legislative assembly district. Lawmakers certainly didn't want to preside over the districts with the "most unhealthy" kids.

By the same token, since organizational leadership is critical in driving change—one decision by an "early adopter" may influence the environments of thousands—advocates should also target employers, documenting the health and productivity improvements from investments in physical activity in the workplace. Leaders at the forefront of change in this area often have a personal stake in health promotion. The superintendent of the Los Angeles Unified School District pushed a districtwide soda ban in 2002 after being diagnosed with type 2 diabetes. President Bill Clinton partnered with the American Heart Association after his heart attack to engage the beverage industry in voluntarily withdrawing sodas from schools. And in Arkansas the governor's substantial weight loss after his diabetes diagnosis and the state House speaker's heart attack precipitated their shepherding legislation to create healthy school environments.

Another way to galvanize grassroots advocacy is to expose inequities in the distribution of public-recreation "goods" in low-income communities, along with overcrowded and outdated schools, supermarket scarcity, and the proliferation of fast-food franchises. Litigation threatened by the City Project persuaded the Los Angeles Unified School District board to adopt regulations to improve the quality of PE for its 700,000 students and increase compliance with state mandates for PE duration. Advocacy has also spurred local public parks and recreation department innovation in modest redevelopment efforts, such as creating "pocket" parks on small vacant urban lots. In West Philadelphia, an effort of this sort was launched to address multiple interests. An architecture class project at University of Pennsylvania that was linked to an urban renewal and redesign effort charged students with equipping recreation areas with durable weather- and vandalism-resistant play and fitness equipment. These areas incorporated green space and were to be located in close proximity to bus stops to enhance the safety of mass transit riders and accessibility to the physical activity space.

Food-Policy Follies and Gym-Policy Gyrations

Thin scientific evidence is often cited to justify inaction on physical activity, but thin science doesn't seem to deter nutrition advocates. Targeting food and nutrition is still the order of the day for obesity- and chronic-disease-control policy. Clinical studies have shown the greater harm of trans fats (those by-products of trying to solidify vegetable oil into margarine) than the saturated fats they replace. Researchers have estimated the number of first-time heart attacks and strokes that could be averted if trans fats were eliminated from the food supply (Willett 2006). Progressive cities like New York have used these studies to persuade city councils to ban trans fats. But no one, to my knowledge, has demonstrated actual health improvements from such bans. It seems likely that restaurateurs and Big Food will just go back to using saturated fats, since no one's come up with another alternative that produces the same taste and texture.

The same exact kind of evidence is available to calculate the protective effects of small amounts of physical activity on chronic-disease rates—and health enhancements far beyond what trans fat bans can accomplish (Physical Activity Guidelines Advisory Committee 2008). Yet skepticism abounds that intervening to reintegrate a few extra minutes of extra physical activity into our daily lives can be feasible or effective. The rational use of credible evidence often seems to be MIA when it comes to obesity policy discussions. Back to the Kersh and Morone article (2002) from one of the premier health policy journals that I use in my class. "The Politics of Obesity: Seven Steps to Government Action" mentions physical activity only once—on the next-to-last page in a passing refer-ence to a 2002 White House fitness initiative. In a bizarre non sequitur in the next and final paragraph, the article asserts that public health advocates perceive government regulation of fatty foods to "constitute necessary protection against 'North Americans' sedentary suicide" (153). There's absolutely no evidence that more expensive or less accessible fatty food launches people out of their seats, nor that public health advocates think it does. The take-home message to me is that a twenty-first-century article on government intervention to address obesity was published in a scholarly journal without any attention to physical activity. It's outra-geous that it passed peer review.

Compounding the situation is the weakness of the few policies to increase physical activity that are getting the most attention. For example, as our study (described in chapter 1) and many others attest, increasing the length of gym class or recess periods won't increase kids' physical activity levels unless they provide the resources to make sure the kids are actually exercising during PE and recess (Morabia and Costanza 2009).

Lessons from Other Social-Change Movements: Left Behind!

The marquee success of twentieth-century public health was tobacco-use prevention and control. While some have argued that policy change precedes social-norm change, history suggests the reverse. The politi-cal will to drive the passage of legislation and the success of litigation occurred *late* in tobacco control, following widespread norm change. California's smoke-free workplace act, passed in 1995 and implemented in 1998, was preceded by years of organizationally imposed smoking bans and subsequent regulatory requirements to maintain smoke-free workplaces. Declines in adult smoking rates began well before the pas-sage of the tobacco excise tax in 1988 (Messer et al. 2007). The primacy of social-norm change may be seen in the greater success of tobacco control in the United States than in Europe. European bureaucratic, "top down" mandates have produced high levels of grassroots resistance and anemic compliance and enforcement; witness Geneva's short-lived ban on smoking in restaurants.

Similarly, new HIV infections among older gay white men have decreased, as have alcohol-involved motor collisions, street and high-way littering, and corporate environmental dumping. Seatbelt and child safety-seat use and breastfeeding are on the rise. But the same gains haven't been seen in communities of color that were last on board in advocacy and policy and in programmatic intervention in most of these public health arenas. At present, the more developed environmental solutions to physical inactivity foster active leisure. They rely on volun-tary participation and speak only to those who have the luxury of time and money. They also assume that the culture places a high value on being active, an assumption that just doesn't wash in communities with many more pressing priorities, like preventing their kids from getting shot, keeping a roof over their heads, and putting food in the fridge. This doesn't bode well for sparking a mass movement.

What we need are sociocultural and physical environmental changes that rely *less* on individual motivation and supportive cultural values. We need to organize changes in policy and practice to give incentives for physical activity. We need to upgrade the physical infrastructure of poor communities. This costs time and money—and tends to be low on the totem pole with so many other critical needs. In addition, as described earlier, underserved communities experience more substantial cultural and economic barriers to physical activity participation. As my mentor and friend Shiriki Kumanyika of the University of Pennsylvania tren-chantly observed, "Without structural changes, individually oriented health promotion may inadvertently increase disparities between the more and less advantaged by only fostering risk reduction among those who find it feasible and affordable."

There are myriad examples in which these cultural and economic barriers come into play. Since arduous hair maintenance routinely keeps many African American women and girls from doing anything that would cause them to sweat, we should make short bouts of activity more accessible and appealing. Posters encouraging stair use in a subur-ban Baltimore mall didn't change blacks' behavior until the poster was changed to feature an African American (Andersen et al. 1998; Andersen et al. 2006). Studies usually don't include sufficiently large samples of these populations to break out the findings by ethnicity, and rarely by ethnicity *and* gender or income. In the case of the stair prompts, the strategy itself was not the problem—it was the marketing of the intervention. By the way, depicting an African American in the poster resulted in increases in stair use among African Americans *and* whites. My colleague on the National Physical Activity Plan Coordinating Committee, Bess Marcus, says she's made the same observation in her efforts to recruit diverse samples of research participants—that whites respond to recruitment ads featuring Latinos, but Latinos don't respond to those featuring whites. People in socioeconomically marginalized populations often tune out the mass media, feeling that they're excluded from most opportunities by virtue of income, class, race, immigration status, or other fairly immutable attributes. Racially or ethnically matched subjects in media materials signal their inclusion—messages intended for them. Affluent whites, generally empowered in American society, require no such signal and are more likely to attend to the message itself to determine its relevance to them.

Making organizational changes is logical and pragmatic, particularly *push* strategies that make physical activity hard to avoid. They increase the likelihood of delivering substantial returns on investment to employers by engaging the more sedentary and overweight population segments that have been overlooked by traditional work-site programs. They also get around such barriers as unsafe and unappealing outdoor surroundings, a lack of access to high-quality produce and recreational facilities, an unwillingness to devote scarce leisure time to activity, and copious perspiration during longer bouts of strenuous exercise. Some, in fact, build upon such cultural assets as the dance tradition extending to middle and older adulthood, and collectivist values.

The private and public sectors need to be involved in different ways. The private sector is better at figuring out how to disseminate innovations than the public sector, and since building a brand is costly, maintaining its viability—which includes making sure workers are at their best—is treated with importance from the outset. But profit making is indifferent to outcomes beyond product sales and value. A government bears the brunt of the inactivity of its population and is better able to develop or identify innovations consistent with the public good. Creative ways of forming public-private partnerships would take advantage of the strengths of each sector, and public health agencies are ideally situated to play the role of convener.

Physical Activity Squares Off against Nutrition

Incorporating physical activity is cheaper and easier in many respects than providing access to nutrient-rich whole foods. In addition, it may not be possible to maintain a healthy weight with most Americans' low activity participation. There is also less controversy, conflict, and stigma surrounding the need for, or the benefits of, physical activity than that surrounding diet and nutrition. "Deep pocket" business interests—for example, sporting goods manufacturers and health clubs—stand to *benefit* from the success of these efforts. In contrast, Big Food—soda manufacturers, fast-food franchises, and processed-food producers and distributors, among others—will suffer a reduction in profits if public health efforts are successful. Overconsumption of water, whole grains, legumes, and fruits and vegetables cannot be induced as readily as can the overconsumption of highly processed products containing sugar, fat, salt, caffeine or, more likely, combinations of the above. It's comical to envision people lining up for platefuls of brown rice, broccoli, and lentils the way they do for Pink's Hot Dogs or In-N-Out Burgers, an image that invariably draws guffaws in my lectures. Also, profit margins are razor thin on fragile and perishable whole foods such as fruits, vegetables, and whole grains. Last, but not least, behavioral economists have found that people tend to be more averse to loss than motivated by gain (Camerer 1999). Framing school health policy as protecting against the loss of PE and recess may have more traction than adding salads and fruit, and certainly more than the positively un-American notion of depriving kids of soda and chips!

As I mentioned in chapter 1, physical exertion has historically been completely intertwined with eating and drinking. That the two must interact for optimal human development and health maintenance is hardly far-fetched. We know that proper cognitive and emotional as well as muscular, bone, and organ development in children requires high levels of physical activity (Physical Activity Guidelines Advisory Committee 2008). Adult brains also require regular physical activity to function optimally, like regulating mood and enhancing cognitive processing.

The notion that physical activity and food and drink intake influence each other may be gaining a bit of traction, but it is still widely underappreciated or ignored outright. This relates to eating, in that staying fit in our obesogenic society takes a lot of self-control. One of my postdocs, who had battled obesity most of her life, lamented that it was difficult for her to get home from UCLA (a trek of just a few miles), without stopping off at several drive-through windows on the busy thoroughfares along the way. Neuroscience is just beginning to identify the ways in which physical activity improves executive functioning (Medina 2008; Ratey and Hagerman 2008), the way we process and respond to information. In his book *The End of Overeating* (2009), Dr. David Kessler, the physician who headed the Food and Drug Administration under Presidents George H. W. Bush and Bill Clinton, underscores the key role of executive control in resisting temptation and strengthening the pursuit of goals other than rewarding ourselves with foods high in salt, sugar, and fat. In fact, a part of the long-standing conundrum of physical activity's central role in weight control—that its effect is larger than the number of calories it burns—may rest in this enhancement of cognitive processing that facilitates goal-oriented behavior beyond the immediate gratification of food. But the only reference I could find to physical activity in Kessler's book was an aside about the temptation of driving past a cherished fast-food outlet en route to the gym. I was more than a little surprised that physical activity was nowhere in his discussion of the etiology of the obesity epidemic or in the "food rehab" Rx for weight management, especially since he was at one time evidently a pretty serious athlete—he was drafted by a Canadian pro football team—so he should know better!

Granted, media coverage of the influence of physical activity on cognition is relatively new, but physical activity's positive effects on emotion and reward centers in the brain, raising the levels of certain chemical signals associated with mood elevation, have long been established. And that in itself is another link, albeit indirect, between physical activity and eating. The antidepressant effect of physical activity may help curb the overeating associated with a depressed mood. Even in highlighting the "French paradox"—the French being thinner than Americans despite a higher dietary fat intake—Kessler pointed to smaller portions, less commercial marketing, and a culture that frowns on snacking and gorging, but completely neglected to mention the higher physical activity levels of the French, mostly because of their complete mass transit system, car-unfriendly city centers, and few buildings under five stories with elevators! Just goes to show you how deep the divide is between the exercise and nutrition-science worlds. The culture clash doesn't help the cause either. Disdain for competitive sports is not uncommon among nutrition professionals, most of whom, not coincidentally, are women. At nutrition conferences, I usually have to shake the trees to find a colleague to join me for a little March Madness—after getting puzzled looks from more than a few! But I have to wade into packed hotel lounges and jockey for position at exercise-science meetings just to be able to see what team's playing. Disdain for nutrient-rich whole foods, especially those not traditionally included in the American diet, is not uncommon in exercise-science circles, most of whose members, not surprisingly, are male former athletes. This culture clash was reflected in a Los Angeles ESPN radio ad that aired in April 2006: "We're the prime rib on a dial full of tofu!"

It's interesting, though, that I know of no credible evidence that the converse is true—that eating healthfully favorably influences physical activity levels in any substantial way. My own anecdotal observations support this. Attendees at public health physical activity and exercise-science meetings are noticeably thinner than those attending public health nutrition meetings. Of course the two groups may differ in other ways as well (youth may be on the side of the exercise scientists), but the parallels are pretty striking to me: since neither healthful eating nor physical activity alone is likely to control weight creep in our obesogenic society, I'd venture to say that more of the people dedicated to activity, professionally and personally, eat better than the healthful eaters exercise. And exercise fetishes net more exercise. But eating fetishes net excess calorie consumption, even if the food's healthy.

The role of nutrition in weight management and obesity control is obviously well established, with clearly defined action steps. But the essential role of physical activity in preventing weight gain and regain, while increasingly evident, is *operationally* underdeveloped (Yancey, Pronk, and Cole 2007). For example, similar to point-of-sale posters and banners to promote purchases of fruits and vegetables, activity prompts may be used to promote stair use and sedentary-product labeling—comparing the calories expended while watching a two-hour movie to those burned while playing softball for that same amount of time. Excise taxes on junk food to allow society to recoup some of the "external" costs to society of 99-cent burgers (like ambulance services for transporting 20-year-olds to the emergency room after a heart attack) could be used as a model for taxing autos to subsidize mass transit. Junk-food restrictions on school vending machines could be translated as restrictions on sedentary video games, for example, requiring as many active games like Dance Dance Revolution as games that exercise only the fingers. But food-focused interventions are more intuitive, because nutrition has been a part of public health policies—pasteurizing milk, preventing water contamination, encouraging breastfeeding—since their inception. Physical activity is a newcomer, and it may provoke resistance from the legions of nutritionists who may view activity promotion as competition for scarce resources, especially in tightening economic circumstances.

SO WHERE DO WE GO FROM HERE?

If we're serious about preventing and controlling obesity and chronic disease, we absolutely must focus our energies on building social cohesion and changing cultural norms to support physical activity. We have to act in concert to generate the political will to make the aggressive changes that will ultimately be necessary for long-term success. Immediate steps include:

1. Influencing decision making by early adopter leaders governing high-exposure settings (work sites, schools, day care centers), especially in the public sector to which the costs and benefits accrue in many areas. One employer, organizational leader, politician, school

principal or board member, minister, talk show host, or foundation or government-agency executive can influence the social environments of hundreds or thousands of people.

2. Developing approaches that work when people don't have much motivation, don't belong to cultures that place a priority on active leisure, don't have a lot of discretionary time or money, and don't have ready access to appealing, well-maintained recreational facilities. These characteristics and constraints are typical of ethnic minority and low-income communities faced with longer commutes, poor-quality child care, and unfavorable attitudes toward exercise born of generations of relegation to manual labor and walking long distances for transportation. Workplace practices and policies instituting brief exercise breaks on paid time or providing substantial mass transit and remote-parking incentives will increase physical activity levels across the entire organization more than on-site gyms for use during discretionary time or lunchtime walking groups. The latter policies are more likely to be utilized by people who are already active and who are generally higher in the workplace hierarchy. The former policies are more likely to be used by less fit staff members, and frankly, saving $50 a month on parking means more to a cafeteria worker than a professor. Policies and practices favoring the sedentary thereby increase overall individual *and* organizational benefits, delivering a return on investment that may spur dissemination to other organizations.

3. Placing a *central* and concerted emphasis on building a robust public health infrastructure for physical activity promotion to coordinate efforts at obesity prevention and control in order to begin to redress physical activity's status as the stepchild of obesity prevention and control, with nutrition as the favored child (Yancey et al. 2007).

Step 3 deserves particular emphasis. At a recent obesity conference, former US surgeon general Dr. David Satcher described physical activity as the most promising preventive strategy in our public health arsenal and also the most underutilized. Restructuring daily life to incorporate physical activity is crucial. People are often blissfully unaware of their poor fitness because so little obligatory physical activity is necessary in postmodern life. Consequently, there is little demand for physical-activity-related goods and services. Primary demand is driven by biological or cultural necessity: hunger, for example, or religious ritual. Secondary demand is created by marketing. While most people are reluctant to admit the influence of ads on their behavior, profit-driven companies would hardly devote a third of their budgets to marketing if it didn't work. An example of the influence of branding is recent research showing that kids report fruits and veggies to be tastier if they are labeled with the McDonald's golden arches than if they are presented generically.

Doing a little social reengineering to reinject obligatory physical activity into daily life is a logical starting point to achieve widespread physical activity improvement. Many of these involve small, "do-able" changes, like incorporating brief activity bouts during the work or school day, pricing parking permits to increase the number of employees choosing remote lots, adjusting elevators to stop on alternate floors, or even grounding elevators during certain times of the day (allowing regular elevator access only for the disabled). These strategies don't cost much money and are well within the decisional latitude of tens of thousands of middle and upper managers, government administrators, elected officials, political appointees, elders or ordained leaders in religious institutions, community advocates and activists, and youth leaders. They are certainly more useful than government-funded media campaigns educating individuals to just move more—cleverly guised Reaganesque "Just say no" messages that do nothing to address the structural impediments to increasing activity.

THREE

The Evolution of an Idea

WHO, EXACTLY, IS TALKING?

You won't recognize me, though I might look vaguely familiar. If you saw me on the street, you'd probably think "athlete" or, maybe, "model." Depending on how I'm dressed, I can fit the stereotype of either: extraordinarily tall, long-limbed, high-cheekboned, almond-eyed, caramel-skinned, rangy but solid. I get stopped in airports for autographs by parents of little girls, eyes searching feverishly to try to figure out which WNBA team is in town. With fifty in my rearview mirror, I last played organized basketball for Northwestern in 1977, so I really can't complain.

I was a born psychiatrist not quite ready to make the final leap separating "shrinks" from "real" docs. I was an articulate and academically sophisticated, yet coltish and unworldly late adolescent not quite ready

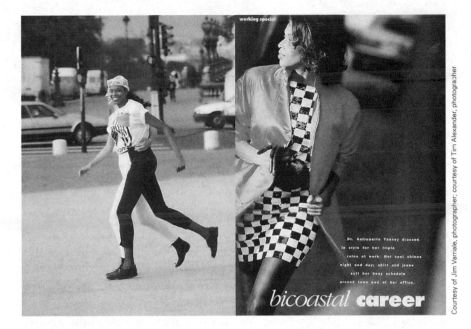

Figure 8.   Pages from the author's portfolio: A test shoot in Paris (1988) and a *Harpers Bazaar* magazine spread (1990).

to plunge into the burdensome adulthood of the practicing physician. I had been too much on track all my life, goal oriented, driven, feeling frivolity and carefree youth slipping too quickly away. And I was the quintessential Don Quixote, determined to show (after all, I'm from just across the river from Missouri, the Show Me State) the elusive *them* (including my ex-husband at the time) who would dare say that I was too tall, too old, too gawky, with too-big feet (11½ AAA) to ever make it in fashion.

So I made it, not onto the covers of *Vogue* or Revlon's billboards, but into the inner chambers of top European designers and fashion photographers and onto the roster of a top Paris agency. I learned an ease of movement in my 6-foot-2-inch frame (still, my mother exercised good judgment in not naming me Grace) and an ease of verbal and nonverbal expression for stage and camera. I also learned a good deal about acting . . . had to learn to finesse it a bit by creating a younger, hip persona . . . intimating that I went to Duke undergrad instead of med school . . . feigning a taste for hip-hop music when I much preferred old-school R&B . . . slogging along club hopping at the likes of the smoky and loud Bain Douche in Paris or the Palladium in New York when I'd rather have been curled up at home with a good book . . . lying a little about my height on my composite card because I *was* too tall and too old—*ancient* by industry standards. (I'd never have gotten my foot in the door if they'd known those stats going in!) And I did all this while practicing thirty to forty hours per week of primary care medicine in mental health centers, ERs, clinics, HMOs, urgent care centers, athletic fields, and foster care agencies in North Carolina, New York, and New Jersey.

Obviously, my modeling career brought me neither fame nor fortune. That wasn't quite what I was after, though I'd have taken it if it had come. I was twenty-four when I walked my first runway before an audience, and twenty-seven when I showed up at my first modeling agency after moving to New York to give it a shot. I was much closer to the ages of the mothers of the teens lining the agency waiting room than I was to my prospective allies and competitors!

In order to walk a runway in Paris, I had to maintain a body weight well below my naturally slim "settling point," then 165 pounds. Getting my weight down to an industry-acceptable level was one of the major obstacles I faced. Dieting, in a conventional sense, was just not something that I could do, not with my scientific training, my athleticism, and the fact that I *felt* and, in fact, *was* slim. So I embarked on a quest, not just to lose weight, but to look and feel the best I possibly could—to beat back Father Time and embrace Mother Earth. I became much more conscientious about getting nutrient "bang" for my calorie "buck." That meant frequenting produce marts, farmers' markets, and health food stores in search of tasty, minimally processed, plant-based foods—heavy on the fruits, vegetables, whole grains, and legumes, light on the fat, sugar, salt, and caffeine. I became an ovo-lacto vegetarian (some eggs, dairy products, and even fish), which helped me make weight at what they called in the business an "athletic 140." Keep in mind that was years before Nike or Adidas started producing active-wear ads for women, so most 6-footers were "hangers" at about 120 pounds—admonished to hang, not fill out, the clothes.

Since then, I've hung up my runway pumps and evolved a different aesthetic for myself—10 extra pounds of upper-body muscle and some lower body weight that's hardly all muscle. My current 175–180 pounds stands me in better stead for the occasional pick-up basketball game with other over-the-hill-gang men and women—I'm definitely ready for my White House invitation! And my cuisine is more quasi-vegetarian than it used to be, since I've developed a lactose intolerance. There are definitely some muscle sags and joint creaks that didn't used to be there. And on the court, I have to make up in savvy what I lack in elevation, playing a more horizontal than vertical game. But I still sometimes get carded trying to buy a six-pack at the corner convenience store, and I very much attribute this, in addition to a favorable genetic endowment, to more than a quarter of a century of scientifically examining the ingredients of a healthy lifestyle and constantly striving to embody and *model* that behavior. Along with recapturing a little *recess* everyday, in work and play.

HOW I FELL IN LOVE WITH PUBLIC HEALTH

My recess model grew out of my experiences in implementing health promotion programs in the '80s and '90s in Los Angeles, New York City, and Richmond, Virginia. I was drawn to preventive medicine and public health because I was regularly reminded of the need to work more upstream—to change organizational, regulatory, and legislative policies. The health of many of the teens I cared for as a general practitioner in foster care agencies was already compromised by some combination of smoking, fast food, sexually transmitted infections, substance abuse, and unintended pregnancy, the latter feeding the cycle of poverty and suboptimal parenting. Many of the adults I saw in community clinics were walking train wrecks, debilitated by diabetes, high blood pressure, heart attacks, and strokes in their forties and fifties. I felt I was treating massive hemorrhaging with band-aids, while most people trudged along, oblivious to the decimation.

It seemed I needed to treat the entire community as a patient, and that wasn't going to happen seeing one person at a time. I noticed that the teens I cared for were puzzled to see a twenty-something woman with no kids and a rewarding and remunerative career—it was outside their limited worldview and made an impression. I started a program for the adolescents in congregate foster care, taking friends and associates to their residential group homes to expose the teens to a variety of role models. Volunteers represented many ethnic backgrounds, ages, shapes and sizes, occupations, vocations, sexual orientation, and family history. Many had experienced some of the same family disruption and dysfunction that led to the teens' placement in foster care. They helped the young people get a realistic idea of how to get from points A to C to Z, as concrete examples of success by hard work and focus, regardless of their starting point.

I continued to manage the program even after I moved to Los Angeles, commuting to New York for a week out of each month. The program ended abruptly when the agency decided that it wasn't really necessary— perhaps they'd found a way to use the program's Medicaid funding to better financial advantage. A colleague at UCLA, Dr. Neal Halfon, later helped me to recognize that I would always risk frustration and disappointment if my focus was on personally delivering a service, rather than advancing the science to drive policy changes mandating the provision of that service. And I'd already come to recognize that doing this kind of work well would require a few more tools in my arsenal. So I went back to school.

I had seen for myself that a little prevention is better than no prevention. And that, since our society has yet to place a high value or priority on prevention, the small amount on offer has to cost little, in time, money, preparation, and effort—to the individual or the organization. I quickly realized that the onus is on public health to create interventions that work under these conditions, and then to convince decision makers of their utility and feasibility.

There was one additional set of experiences that framed my outlook on health promotion. I'd actually moved to New York in the first place to pursue my brief fling with fashion modeling. I had left my psychiatric residency at Duke halfway through, after it dawned on me that I was more interested in mental health and well-being than mental illness. Going to auditions and "go-sees" by day, and working in packed clinics and ERs on nights and weekends, I was struck by the stark contrast between the health education materials we distributed (brochures, fact sheets explaining treatments, and fliers publicizing health fairs or lectures) and the commercial ads that pushed mostly behaviors hazardous to one's health (tobacco, liquor, fast food, and sodas). The former were mostly on white paper, crammed with small black type in a standard font, with dry stats, prescriptions, and dire warnings. The latter were glossy and colorful, with simple and succinct messages. They had well-designed layouts drawing the eye to the central message, hitched to popular cultural icons, with a generous dose of sexual seduction for good measure. Our messages sold our products as a way to fend off death and destruction, while theirs cast their products as spicing up people's already exciting lives. Our approach to getting and keeping the attention of the people we were trying to serve was ass-backward!

A MOSAIC OF LENSES

My first systems-change intervention was my UCLA residency training project in cancer control. My colleagues and I produced culturally targeted patient education docudramas with music and vivid street scenes in English and Spanish promoting mammograms and Pap smears for low-income women seen at public clinics in Los Angeles County. The project was added to a large federally funded Division of Cancer Control study to provide these cancer-screening services to middle-aged and older women seeking care at county clinics for other chronic conditions such as hypertension or diabetes. Having practiced in similar clinic settings in New York City, I had firsthand experience of the difficulties imposed by heavy patient loads and limited translation and medical staffing assistance and equipment. Through patient education videos running in waiting rooms, intervention delivery was intended to be integral to clinic operations without increasing staff burden. The video loop lasted 60 minutes and automatically repeated; the registration desk clerk only had to start it at the beginning of the day, and stop it at day's end.

We were concerned that the staff would become irritated by the repetitive sound and neglect to use the tapes. To the contrary, we found that the videos helped the clerks by decreasing patient complaints about waiting time and demands for information or immediate service. The lesson from the success of the intervention in increasing Pap smear screening rates came through loud and clear: an unobtrusive and practical intervention that resonates culturally with the end-user or targeted group, requires minimal ongoing investment by the implementing organization, and serves a purpose for that organization can be both effective and sustainable.

Because the design of the main study had been set before I joined the division, my add-on intervention could not be independently evaluated in that context. I received a small supplementary award from the funder to test the videos at a community health center in New York where I had worked as a general practitioner, as well as at a free clinic in Venice, California, with which UCLA was associated. We were able to show that the number of Pap smears increased significantly among patients receiving care during the weeks the videos were playing. Another key finding came from the success of the videos on both coasts: their appropriateness for a heterogeneous sample of Latinas, one predominantly of Caribbean Island descent, and the other mostly of Mexican or Central American heritage. This validated our inclusive video production approach for the Spanish-language video. Rather than treat this population as monolithic, we deliberately recruited subjects from a variety of backgrounds (Argentinean, Mexican, Salvadoran) to complement the Puerto Rican narrator, and we chose Latin music of cross-national popularity.

My supplementary award then allowed me to pursue my true calling—promoting physical activity and healthful eating. Dr. Les Breslow, my mentor who was the lead investigator on the larger study, sparked my twenty-year partnership with social psychologist Bill McCarthy by connecting us as energetic young investigators both outside the mainstream of cancer control. At that time, the field was focused on finding a pill to deliver the plant-derived nutrients to prevent cancer, while Bill and I had independently arrived at the "whole foods" approach that is now mainstream. Bill was also a passionate marathon runner, so we teamed up to pursue nutrition- and fitness-intervention research projects, with Bill as the detail-oriented idealist and methodologist, and me as the pragmatic, "big picture" innovator.

I have to pause here to emphasize how important it is to have a mentor, preferably a visionary like Les. He read every memo, report, article, and video script I wrote during my residency and beyond, and got back to me in a few days with extensive comments and recommendations. This from a man who was revered in the field as a pioneer, the modern father of public health. He headed several large studies and was on national and international committees that had him crisscrossing the world more than I now do this country. He taught me what can't be learned from books or in the classroom. He also provided a concrete example of how to get it done and, sometimes more importantly, what to get done, when to do it, and whom to engage in the effort. He met my father once at a little dinner party I hosted for my parents when they were in town. Turned out he and my dad were both World War II vets who'd been on Okinawa at the same time. They traded a few war stories, but it's doubtful that they'd met—Les was a commissioned officer and doctor tracking down parasites, and my dad was a noncommissioned staff sergeant on the front lines. However, they were less than a year apart in age, and it was clear they shared many similar perspectives. My dad's been gone now for nearly two decades, but that experience allows me to recapture a little of my father's spirit in Les. Perhaps, for that reason, the lessons Les has taught me as my mentor surface in my poetry. Or maybe he inhabits that most intimate space because of the indomitable spirit he shares with others I've long admired from afar—Martin, Malcolm, Shirley, Barbara, Audre, JFK, Jimmy, and Bill. Having had an opportunity to observe him engage with "paupers" and "kings," I can attest to his treatment of all with respect and appreciation for their humanity, abilities, and contributions. I can also attest to his refusal to accept anything less than the best, from others (like me!) and, particularly, from himself.

Les opened the door for me to spend a little time during the last part of my preventive medicine residency at the Cooper Institute for Aerobics Research. Hanging out at the place the American fitness craze started—the largest and oldest non-university exercise research center

Did You Ever Have a Mentor?

Did you ever have a mentor?
The question came to me
Because I have the best
And his *name* is Les

Did someone ever see you
In a way no other has?
See *you* as supremely able?
Having a place at every table

Did someone ever teach you
About wielding power in a way
That focuses on the mission
And leaves egos to go fishin'?

Did someone ever give you
That ultimate resource so freely
Because time is always precious
Its passing ever more conscious

Did someone ever guide you
In charting out a course?

Show such belief in your ability
That he doled out praise quite
    stingily?

Did someone ever reach you
To let you know the score?
Quietly convey you're off the mark
When others might let you chase
    that lark?

Did someone ever allow you
To grow and evolve unfettered?
In surrounds quite loving
Shared passion always
    forthcoming

Did you ever have a mentor?
Friend, guide, torch carrier?
Hero, beacon, companion?
Emanation of spirit?
Walking here with us!
                T___˙ (March 17, 2005)

in the world, founded by the doc who coined the term *aerobics*, was exhilarating. My training there not only expanded my skill set and my professional network, but it also offered a history lesson.

A HISTORICAL PERSPECTIVE

A movement was born in the mid-twentieth century, built on the work of Kenneth Cooper. Dr. Cooper is a pioneer in the field of preventive medicine. An aspiring astronaut, he joined the Army as a physician in 1957, the year I was born. He then transferred to the Air Force and worked with NASA to improve astronauts' physical conditioning for space travel. He returned to school to earn his master's degree in public health and wound up doing the work that heralded the formal study of exercise as good medicine. He helped to move the scientific view of battling disease and enhancing and restoring health through lifestyle change from the margins to the mainstream . . . and it started with autopsies. Dr. Cooper saw that the severity of coronary artery blockage he found among Vietnam War casualties at autopsy was directly linked to how these soldiers had performed on the fitness tests they were subjected to as soldiers. The better their performance, the cleaner their arteries at the time of autopsy. He invented a fitness concept based on his research and introduced it to the world in the title of his 1968 bestseller, *Aerobics*. In the preface to his third book, *The New Aerobics* (1970, 5), he wrote:

> When I introduced aerobics as a new concept of exercise, my chief aim was to counteract the problems of lethargy and inactivity which are so widely prevalent in our American population. Therefore, my first book was mainly a motivational book, but also it was an attempt to encourage people to examine more closely the benefits to be gained from regular exercise. The wide public acceptance of *Aerobics* indicates that these objectives have been at least partially achieved.

Dr. Cooper gradually built a critical mass of medical, business, and public health leaders who were similarly convinced of the major contribution of physical activity and other daily habits to health and longevity. These leaders included Les, who was on the institute's advisory board. Apparently they were right, because Les turned ninety-four in 2009 and still comes to the office three or four times a week. Ken's pushing eighty and still runs the institute.

The strategy, which seems obvious now, was to increase leisure time physical activity—back then mostly jogging—to improve cardio-respiratory or *aerobic* fitness, spurred by knowledge of cardiovascular disease risks and prevention. Aerobics is now common in the lay and health-professional vernacular. The range of activities promoting aerobic fitness has evolved over time, but many people, particularly younger, affluent white men, continue the running or jogging tradition.

Dr. Cooper's *Aerobics*, which popularized the fitness trend, was intended as individual advice based on military conditioning routines, and indeed, engaging in leisure time physical activity for the express purpose of improving fitness was revolutionary for the time. His influence and activism increased the number of American joggers from a hundred thousand in 1968 to 30 million today. Dr. Cooper was right that his work helped a large segment of the public to understand, as he writes, the benefits of regular exercise. But unfortunately, neither that book, nor the myriad titles (nearly 30,000 Amazon.com listings) that have followed his tradition have mobilized the majority of the population to do what they know they should do.

LAUNCHING MY LIFE'S WORK

In recruiting for the gym-based pilot study I proposed to the funder in my supplementary grant application during my residency, I sent out a press release to most Los Angeles news outlets. Much to my surprise, a health reporter from the *Los Angeles Times* responded. The resulting story, "A Medical Imbalance," took up most of the front page of a weekday Life & Style section, complete with this photo of several pilot study participants and me. Talk about a picture being worth a thousand words! The photo and the article, which addressed the low levels of participation of African American women in public health research, generated a thousand phone calls from prospective participants. The pilot study ended up with 429 subjects, more than in the full-scale study that was funded several years later. I had to quickly borrow $10,000 in research funding from my very generous colleague, Dr. Susan Love (who was running the breast cancer center at UCLA at the time), just to be able to collect data from all of the women clamoring to participate.

That was my first real experience with marketing, and one of the best things to come out of it was my now nearly two-decade collaboration and friendship with Octavia Miles, an MBA and former Mattel Toys marketing exec. Octavia called me three times in response to the *Times* article. The third message she left was a terse, "Dr. Yancey, I am *not* accustomed to having my phone calls ignored. You *must* need some help. Call me as soon as possible!" Which I did immediately upon retrieving the message, and the rest, as they say, is history. Best decision I ever

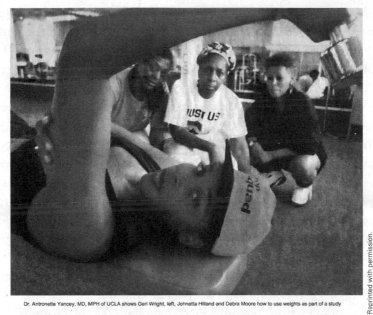

Dr. Antronette Yancey, MD, MPH of UCLA shows Geri Wright, left, Johnetta Hilland and Debra Moore how to use weights as part of a study

November 01, 1994
SHARI ROAN, TIMES
HEALTH WRITER

A Medical Imbalance

After a long history of testing treatments primarily on white men, scientists are trying to include women and minorities. Attracting them could mean saving more lives--but it's a challenge

It was envisioned as one of the first ethnically balanced, large-scale studies of its kind: a trial of 16,000 women to test tamoxifen's ability to prevent breast cancer in women at high risk.

But when researchers began recruiting subjects for the nationwide drug study in 1992, they were able to attract few minorities. Just 2% of the initial study population were African Americans, Asian Americans, Latinas or Pacific Islanders.

A later recruiting drive, this time targeting ethnic groups, raised the percentage to 4. But researchers, who had hoped for up to 20%, remain troubled. If a significant number of minority women aren't enrolled soon, researchers will be unable to answer a key question when the study ends: Does the drug work any differently in women of color?

Experts now estimate that about 60% of the study's final 5,000 to 6,000 women will have

to be minorities--a daunting number by any research standards--in order to answer that question.

Researchers in the tamoxifen study are hardly alone in their dilemma. After a long history of testing medical treatments primarily on white men, scientists performing federally funded research are now generally required to enroll a certain percentage of women in the studies and, in many cases, a certain percentage of racial minorities.

But opening this door to better and certainly more equitable science has

not resulted in a flood of candidates. Many studies designed to include minority women are sorely lacking in participants.

"Almost all the studies going on right now are underrepresented in terms of women of color," says Dr. Antronette K. Yancey, an assistant professor of public health at UCLA.

The reasons for the poor participation are complex and suggest that improvements won't be simple to achieve. According to Dr. Machelle Allen, an obstetrician at the New York University Medical Center who has studied the issue, the reasons include:

* a history of unethical and abusive studies involving minority groups;

* discrimination in medical care;

* practical barriers, such as a lack of transportation to clinical trials or time to participate in them.

According to an article by Allen in a recent issue of the Journal of the American Medical

Figure 9. After being featured in the *Los Angeles Times*'s Life & Style section in an article addressing the paltry numbers of African American women in public health research, Dr. Yancey's gym-based pilot study swelled from thirty to more than four hundred participants.

made, because Octavia thought completely differently than my scientist colleagues, a perfect foil to their caution and observance of convention. As a bonus, then–State Senator Diane Watson, now recently retired as a US congresswoman, saw the article and signed up in a show of support.

In the midst of this experience and with the growing recognition that you can reach many more of the people in greatest need of preventive services if you offer those services to "captive audiences," I agreed to take over a fitness project that was threatened with losing its funding at Charles Drew University, a medical school in southern Los Angeles. I immediately hired Octavia, who'd become my right hand as a volunteer on my pilot study at the gym ever since I called her back. The project was part of a state-run, federally funded initiative charged with engaging residents of nine ethnic minority communities in regular physical activity. Rather than host exercise classes at Drew, we branched out to provide free on-site fitness instruction in nearly fifty community-based organizations concentrated in the areas around Drew.

I'd considered the sites only as convenient staging grounds at the outset of the Drew project, but soon came to appreciate the importance of organizational infrastructure to our ability to get people to participate in the exercise sessions. Like most people who get the idea to start an exercise program, I figured the convenience and camaraderie of the organization was sufficient motivation. Unfortunately, people get real excited at first, and then life gets in the way. Everyone tries to reinvent the wheel, but it always comes out the same. *It comes down to most people's unwillingness to go out of their way to be active.* Physical activity programs are rarely successfully institutionalized; most wither on the vine, die soon after starting, or never get off the ground in the first place. As I worked on the Drew project, it became apparent to me that organizational behavior had a greater influence on the viability of the programs than did the individuals' commitment to be active. The project flourished at the Compton, California, church where the minister himself opened the doors for the exercise classes on Saturdays and, from the pulpit, praised the dedication of, or the results achieved by, participating members. In contrast, attendance dwindled at a nearby church with engaged parishioners but little evidence of leadership commitment—locked exterior doors or equipment cabinets not infrequently resulted in our leading walking groups outdoors rather than aerobic sessions inside the church.

Among our Drew project sites, the organizational characteristic that distinguished those that managed to continue the physical activity beyond the grant period from those that didn't was the utilization of preexisting group cohesiveness and support (Yancey, Miles, and Jordan 1999). Most other characteristics associated with the institutionalization of public health programs were present across all the organizations—an aggressive "in-group" program champion, large captive audiences, site leadership commitment, preexisting mechanisms for regular communication within the site such as newsletters or announcement periods, an alignment of mission, and an established productive relationship with the implementing agency (in this case Charles Drew University)—probably because the program would not have been adopted in their absence.

I moved to Richmond, Virginia, on the heels of the Drew project, to accept the position of the city's director of public health. There I was charged with bringing the department into the twenty-first century, where chronic diseases kill or disable the majority of people. I devoted a lot of my energy as well as political capital to organizing the delivery of exercise instruction by launching the Rock! Richmond campaign. There were several strategies to accomplish this: (1) providing free memberships to community health and fitness clubs; (2) deploying fitness instructors to community sites like churches, senior centers, and nonprofit agency offices; and (3) training lay fitness instructors (akin to lay health advisers). The sessions were convenient (located near home, work, or worship) and low cost (free to $3 per session), and the incentives were popular. For example, "Rock dollars" were distributed at the end of each exercise session, redeemable for fitness-promoting branded merchandise like pedometers, water bottles, and baseball caps. Regardless, people began with the best of intentions, but participation fell off dramatically after the first few months. Only the die-hards remained after a few months—mostly those who were already availing themselves of many other fitness options! On the upside, though, participants at the Rock! Richmond sites were at a higher risk for chronic disease than the general public (Yancey et al. 2003) and undoubtedly at a higher risk than most people utilizing private fitness facilities.

One of the best moves I made in Richmond was my first hire there, Todd Berrien, an old friend from my New York days who was a graphic designer, fine artist, and former creative director at Frasier Smith, a Saatchi & Saatchi ad agency. He had created the Miller Brewing Co. Sound Express ad campaign for which I'd been hired as a model, though neither of us knew it until the proofs from the photo shoot came back. Todd became, as far as I know, the first social marketing director at a local health department, at a time when I was just beginning to understand the concept. His is the creative genius that brought my 3 a.m. brainstorms to life—with a vengeance—along with coming up with a few of his own, like challenging the city to break the record for the largest group exercise session and putting the mayor on an exercise machine in City Council chambers to launch Rock! Richmond. You might wonder how I persuaded a six-figure-salaried, high-flying ad agency exec to take a big pay cut and join the minions slaving away in obscurity, buried in a government bureaucracy. It wasn't the job security. I just knew from a lot of lunches and happy hours that Todd was a vegan Buddhist who felt he was in serious need of a karmic overhaul. (Todd's Upper West Side office in New York was just across the street from the doc-in-the-box clinical practice where I worked, and we met when he brought his daughter in as a patient.) Ours has become a quarter-century creative collaboration and a great friendship. We published a coffee table book of poetry and art in 1997, *An Old Soul with a Young Spirit*, that sold out its first edition (albeit only 2,000 copies). I was best person in his wedding in Martha's Vineyard, along with his longtime buddy as best man and his son as his "main man" (the title of one of his paintings of his son as a child). I think it's fair to say that regardless of what brought Todd to public health, it's now a match made in heaven.

In launching Rock! Richmond, we were most interested in conveying the message that *everyone*, heavy and lean, black and white, young and old, male and female, could and should be physically active. The mayor, a reluctant participant at best, was railroaded into being supportive by his wife—one of our staunchest advocates. She'd lost about 30 pounds and was a true convert. She got that it was not just about educating individuals to change but pushing the cultural envelope. So she helped

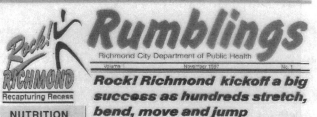

Rumblings

Richmond City Department of Public Health

Volume 1 — November 1997 — No. 1

Rock! Richmond
Recapturing Recess

Rock! Richmond kickoff a big success as hundreds stretch, bend, move and jump

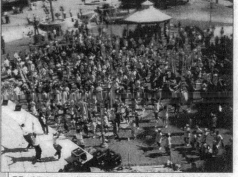

NUTRITION

Antioxidants

If you peel a banana or an apple and leave it out in the air, it will soon begin to turn brown. This process is called oxidation and is the result of oxygen inter-acting with the fruit and breaking it down. Oxygen and other com-pounds can have the same effects inside our body. Fortunately the breakdown is not as fast as the banana or apple, but over 20 - 30 years, it can have a significant effect. Several leading medical authorities believe that many dis-eases, including several types of cancer, are related to this oxidation process.

The good news is there is a way to slow this process and it does not cost a fortune. Several foods contain vit-amins and minerals that serve as antioxidants. Antioxidants will interact

(Continued on page 2)

Hopefully by now you have heard about Rock! Richmond. This program, spon-sored by the Richmond City Department of Public Health, aims to increase physical activity and healthy eating in the lives of the city's citizens. You might wonder why we are taking on such a project. Public health departments were first formed to fight the epidemics of infectious diseases such as TB and cholera. As we look forward to the 21st Century, we are facing a new epidemic - becoming couch potatoes. Only about 37% of the citizens in Richmond exercise on a regular basis. As a result, the majority of our citizens have a greater risk of developing a "lifestyle" disease. For instance, diabetes has increased dramatically over the past 14 years,

especially among the African-American pop-ulation. This can be traced to two facts — we are less active and are fatter than our ances-tors. High blood pressure, strokes, heart dis-ease, colon cancer, and even breast cancer can be related to too little activity and poor eating habits. You can decrease your odds of developing these diseases if you become more physically active and eat properly.

There are 31 Rock! Richmond sites offering FREE exercise classes, including nutrition education. We are also seeking additional sites for these exciting classes. Call 608-3175 to locate the site closest to you or if you are interested in starting a site of your own with at least ten other city residents.

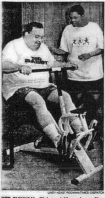

GET PHYSICAL. Richmond Mayor Larry Cha-vis gets training pointers from city Depart-ment of Public Health Director Dr. Antronette K. Yancey. His T-shirt says, "Big Daddy."

Richmond mayor rocks world of physical fitness

Official uses weight of office to kick off health campaign

BY GORDON HICKEY
TIMES-DISPATCH STAFF WRITER

First he did the Macarena, and now he's plunked himself on a "sport trainer" — a sort of bucking exercycle — for all the world to see. Can bungee jumping be very far in the future for Richmond Mayor Larry E. Chavis?

In January, Chavis and other members of the City Council did the Macarena in support of the United Negro College Fund's benefit. Yesterday, Chavis kicked off the Rock Richmond physical fitness campaign by donning a "Big Daddy" T-shirt and doing a few stationary laps outside his second-floor City Hall office.

The point of yesterday's public relations event was "to gather the city behind physical fitness," Chavis said. "All of us need to be more active, particularly myself."

Chavis, who is the definition of XXL, said he has lost as much as 100 pounds in the past but has always put the weight back on. "This time I'm going to pace myself. It's a lifelong process," he said.

Rock Richmond was developed by city De-partment of Public Health Director Dr. Antron-ette K. Yancey.

She pointed out that "most people who die in the city die from chronic disease. . . . Rock Rich-mond is aimed at increasing people's activity and nutritious eating."

She said the Rock Richmond staff will work with groups and organizations such as churches and will mount a media campaign to support healthy living. They also will work with city employees, who number more than 4,000. Yan-cey said the particular focus will be on the Police Department.

She said the physical fitness campaign also can reduce crime because if people are out on the streets participating in healthy activities like walking, criminals will be more likely to stay out of sight.

She also said that a healthy work force has fewer sick days and is more productive. "We can be a better city if people are at home fewer days," she said.

Yesterday, Chavis did a complete workout, including warm-up, stretching, aerobic time on the sports rider and a session of weight lifting. While that kicked off the public relations cam-paign, the official start of Rock Richmond is set for Oct. 2.

On that day, Yancey said, she hopes the city will set a world record for the largest number of people in a group exercising at the same time. The event is scheduled for Nina F. Abady Festi-val Park between the Coliseum and 6th Street Marketplace.

Courtesy of the *Richmond Times-Dispatch*; courtesy of Todd Berrien, graphic designer

Figure 10. Getting the city of Richmond moving and rockin'—starting with the mayor.

change the menus for the closed City Council chamber meetings with department heads, got us into the main foyer of City Hall for our Friday lunchtime aerobics sessions, and otherwise served as an insider facilitator to everything we were trying to do!

When I left for Richmond, the full-scale cancer prevention study, Fighting Cancer with Fitness (FCF), that Bill McCarthy and I had developed from our pilot findings, had just been funded. Fortunately, Bill and other colleagues like Joanne Leslie stepped up, with Octavia Miles leading the charge, doing the "up close and personal" work of the study in my absence. In a nutshell, FCF was a randomized controlled trial involving 360 middle- and working-class African American women in which all participants were given a free one-year membership to the health club study site. Experimental group participants were instructed in healthy food preparation and selection, and supervised in the use of the gym equipment. Control participants discussed cancer screening, tobacco control, menopause, and other women's health topics of their choosing. Experimental and control classes met weekly for two hours on alternate days of the week, and we followed the women for one year. As with most physical activity trials, the FCF educational intervention in that study was most effective only in the short term (Yancey, McCarthy, et al. 2006). In the long run, women in the control group who'd had to figure out for themselves how best to change their lives and utilize their gym memberships were better able to sustain the changes than were the participants to whom we provided 16 hours of training in use of the fitness equipment and how to fit in physical activity and healthy eating. One thing became clear—if free memberships resulted in only modest changes, subsidies (as in discounted membership fees offered by many health insurance companies) were not likely to produce meaningful change. This underscored a point I'd encountered repeatedly—people who go out of their way to work up a sweat on their own time are different from most folks: they're already fairly active. The question remained, How do we move the *masses*?

When I was recruited back to Los Angeles to develop the county health department's Chronic Disease Prevention and Health Promotion Division, the sheer size and diversity of the catchment area (a population of 10 million with more languages spoken than in any other US locale) required different tactics and approaches. These differences were compounded by the repeated demonstrations of the lack of sustainability of prior approaches, and by the relative resource constraints. (I got about $1 per capita in Richmond, a city of 200,000 and a metropolitan statistical area of less than 1 million; but we had proportionately much, much less to work with in Los Angeles County.)

The challenge for our new division was to design low-cost interventions targeting sedentary women and ethnic minority populations from poor neighborhoods, while improving the overall health of the county. Of course, I'd brought my social marketing guru, Todd, with me, so I was already ahead of most health departments but still lagged far behind the deep-pocket industries exploiting our biological vulnerabilities, which hit marginalized populations hardest. The necessity of community engagement had been reinforced by my earlier work, and I remembered the many settings we used: nonprofit social services agencies, civic groups, public housing developments, local government programs and departments, small businesses, churches, clinics, schools, substance abuse treatment centers, recreation centers, and shopping malls.

Meantime, revised recommendations from the Centers for Disease Control and Prevention and the American College of Sports Medicine were gaining traction. They suggested alternatives to the then-standard 20 minutes of continuous vigorous exercise three days per week. Instead, longer durations of moderate-intensity physical activity performed more regularly (five or more days a week), and exercise sessions broken up into shorter (at least 10-minute) bouts. In conceptualizing a strategy that could take advantage of the new recommendations, I thought about dance, which everyone except curmudgeons views positively. So why not get people up and having fun and moving together to music for short intervals before they even realized they were exercising? These short breaks could fit into the regular routine in settings in which people (captive audiences) spent a lot of time for a variety of purposes—work, worship, learning, socializing, planning, and organizing—with the music and moves adapted for different settings and cultural groups. I hired an exercise physiologist to help me structure the movements so that people who weren't particularly fit or agile wouldn't hurt themselves. I started leading these breaks most every time I lectured or attended a meeting.

Most people seemed to like them, although some skated out the back door when they saw me coming. People got accustomed to them and even complained when the breaks *didn't* happen. People began requesting diagrams and tapes of the moves. My boss at the time, Dr. Jonathan Fielding, went along with the idea (a lot of these were *his* meetings), but insisted that I start gathering data to evaluate the breaks. That was the birth of the *Lift Off!*, or *Lift* those buns *Off* the couches and chairs!

AN EMERGING PERSPECTIVE

The stars must have been aligned in 1999. Elena Subirats, a staff health educator and former athlete at the national Mexican Ministry of Health in Mexico City (Mexico's equivalent to the Centers for Disease Control and Prevention), and Bill Kohl, a colleague whom I met during my residency rotation days at the Cooper Institute, came up with similar ideas in the same time period. Bill developed *Take 10!* for the International Life Sciences Institute in Atlanta, engaging elementary school students in 10-minute exercise lessons integrated into their academic curriculum (kindergartners counting while doing a military march). *Pausa para tu Salud* (Pause for Your Health) was virtually identical to the recess-model component of our division's *Fuel Up/Lift Off! LA* social marketing campaign. Of course, we didn't find out about each other's work until years later.

As we introduced *Lift Off!* more broadly, the resonance of certain cultural factors in communities of color was further reinforced; these included family- and community-centered activities, the church as a political and social as well as religious institution and, of course, the importance of music and dance. We were frequently reminded that these types of interventions are institutionalized in other countries such as Japan—in corporations, mass media, supermarkets, and schools. Not to mention Italian immigrant chefs caught on camera starting their workday with group stretches.

Our target groups' high rates of inactivity demanded an intervention approach that could *active*-ate unfit and overweight folks not very far

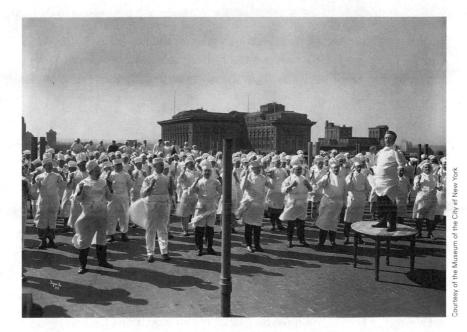

Courtesy of the Museum of the City of New York

Figure 11. The benefit of a fit and healthy workforce is not a new concept. Our *Lift Off!* campaign has frequently been compared to international exercise institutionalization practices such as Chef Leoni leading his cooks in exercise in 1920s New York City, reflecting his Italian roots.

along the path toward adopting fit lifestyles (if they'd even found the path). First, they needed to feel competent. Unlike eating—not terribly challenging for most—dance involves movement skills coming into *play*. And a lot of these folks had been on the short end of the stick in childhood games, with some pretty bad memories of being taunted, teased, or excluded.

But at the same time, the approach also had to excite and motivate people with a range of fitness levels, athleticism, and functional abilities, including exercise buffs and gym rats who might help "carry the water" in pushing for and implementing such changes. One way to do this was to weave in specific dance movements and rhythms, sports traditions, and activity-linked themes and icons with cultural resonance. Another was to invoke the notion of these breaks as an entitlement—the way many people feel about coffee or smoking breaks. After all, most active people don't get as much exercise as they want or feel they need. Of course, there are the naysayers—the holier-than-thou types that run or lift everyday and dismiss such modest amounts of activity as a waste of time.

INSPIRATION—THE ART AND SCIENCE BEHIND THE RECESS MODEL

The scientific innovation of the recess model is its exploitation of the socio-cultural environment to achieve broad reach and penetration. Through social controls like social norms and peer pressure, social support, and organizational self-interest, recess breaks may deliver a small "dose" to the majority, rather than a large dose to a small minority. Unlike most interventions, which deliver the greatest benefits to those who are already active, recess breaks are most beneficial to the least active and fit.

When one of my current doctoral students, Jammie Hopkins, first joined our team as an intern, he asked for my advice in selecting his kinesiology master's thesis project. He was quite an accomplished dancer and choreographer and wanted to see whether he could increase participation at a local community center by offering an African dance class. I suggested that he consider simplifying the moves and packaging it as a 10-minute exercise break. I asked him to estimate how many people he could expose to African dance with a class offered weekly at one community location, compared with all of the work sites, churches, and schools regionally and nationally that would see it and might adopt it as a part of their regular routine. Especially when his intent was to get sedentary and unfit people moving—people who'd never darken the door of an exercise facility. So Jammie got on board and is now the principal choreographer of our *Instant Recess* breaks. His *African Dance Lift Off!* DVD is one of our most popular and has been purchased by organizations in most states. He's also the lead intervention specialist on our federally funded study of *Instant Recess*, the WORKING project.

This took me back to the time when I was asked by the national YMCA to consult on its Gulick Project to revamp the Y's approach and engage a greater proportion of the communities it served. I broached the concept of "Ys Without Walls," in which the Y would expand its business model to contract with employers to provide off-site fitness instruction at the workplace on a weekly or biweekly basis and train internal "wellness coordinators" to lead and champion these activities regularly (at least daily) throughout the week. I understand that the Y is more actively pursuing partnerships with corporations to deliver fitness services on-site now, though to my knowledge, companies are providing personal training and classes on discretionary time rather than weaving the activity into the organizational fabric. I haven't given up, though. I've gotten another of my doctoral students, Catherine Duda, intrigued enough to flesh out the business concept in a couple of her class research papers and pitch it to the managers at a chain fitness club where she works as a part-time trainer.

Recess breaks are not as likely to attract certain active individuals, those in powerful positions who travel frequently and are tethered to their teleconferences and webinars during the limited time they do spend in the office. But it's not just because of inconvenience. The most reluctant participants—sometimes outright resistant to and disparaging of the idea—tend to be white affluent men who'd prefer to jog on their own or compete in sports and don't really get why everyone won't "just do it." Joni Eisenberg, who hosts a radio health talk show for WPFW, the Pacifica affiliate in DC, and also works for the local health department, introduced one of the *Lift Off!* DVDs at an all-staff meeting. The only attendee who was sittin' and snarlin' rather than movin' and shakin' was an older physician who fit that description to a tee. Recess breaks are just not their culture—this strategy is instead tailor-made for women and people of color. In fact, one scientific article noted that "brief [individually performed, discretionary] stretching exercises are more likely to be accepted in Western workplaces, as compared to 'group calisthenics' such as those that have been used in some Japanese workplaces" (Carter and Banister 1994).

But it's OK that there's no one-size-fits-all—there are ways to reintegrate physical activity into daily life that may be more appealing for this demographic. A prime example is a "walk or step while you work" strategy being developed for sedentary office workers by Jim Levine and his team at the Mayo Clinic (Levine and Yeager 2009). Mini stair climbers or bike pedals are placed under the desk, or a standing desk is constructed over a treadmill to permit slow but steady movement. For right now, though, these hybrid strategies that make it easier but not *easy* to make the active choice are definitely the icing, not the cake. A shift in sociocultural norms will still be required to achieve a substantial uptake of this intervention approach, as Levine acknowledged: "We recognize that such an approach must embrace behavioral strategies to affect a sustained intervention and that this . . . can only succeed in increasing daily activity levels with the support of employers" (Levine and Miller 2007). Working-class white men, who are also moving a lot less and gaining girth around the middle, are not especially likely to be found in board rooms or behind desks. Even if they were, *how* to get them to push the pedals and exert themselves, however modestly, is the sticking point. While they may also disdain group dance-type activity, jogging is probably as foreign to them as it is to lower-income Latinos and African Americans. Several of the corporations profiled in chapter 6 that have institutionalized structured group exercise breaks on paid time have predominantly blue-collar white male employees, so clearly the recess approach can be successfully adapted for this group. I'll get into all of this more in the next chapter, on social marketing.

Another central feature of the recess model is its attention to the entire spectrum of factors influencing activity, from biology to geography to economics. Most interventions operate psychologically to motivate behavioral change. Getting sedentary overweight folks to move in order to conform to social norms gets us beyond reliance on personal motivation and volition. It adds biological reinforcement to the psychological motivation, because early in an exercise bout, negative sensations (like fatigue) are outweighed by positive ones (uplifted mood, energy). Feelings of well-being are enhanced and depressive thoughts are dampened by the modest intensity and short duration of the "recess" activity. The social interaction is enjoyable—being "in it together" and engaged on a more human emotional level that momentarily flattens out the workplace hierarchy and puts everyone on equal *foot*ing. But if you're an overweight couch lover, the socializing and positive emotion is

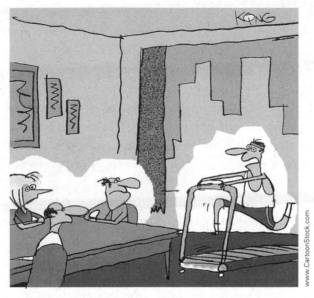

"If I have to be at these boring meetings, I might as well get something out of it."

Figure 12.   Our culture loves to multitask, so why not find a variety of ways to introduce exercise into your daily routine?

accompanied by a physiological reminder—that you've gotten a bit out of shape. You're a bit, or a lot, more out of breath than you would have anticipated from such light exertion! It erodes denial and complacency, creating a little cognitive dissonance for people who typically go about their daily routines needing very little movement, folks who are rarely if ever confronted by the reality of their unfit condition. A typical comment halfway through a 10-minute break is "You mean it's only been five minutes?!!"

Recess breaks not only offer a mechanism for bolstering waxing and waning individual motivation and volition, they also help to circumvent economic constraints and cultural norms that crowd out active leisure. They can be done indoors when outdoor surroundings are not safe or appealing. They don't require special equipment or much space. Don't require an extra bus ride or eat into the precious little time with the kids between long work hours and commutes. Don't mess up the 'do with heavy sweating.

Seduction and persuasion go hand in hand to influence behavior—that's where the art comes in. Corporations know this and invest a big chunk of their budgets on marketing to compete for attention in a very crowded informational environment. The best science is useless in improving the public's health if its cognitive appeals fall on deaf ears, blind eyes, and hard hearts. We have to engage people emotionally as well as intellectually.

People are voting with their feet in demonstrating their resistance to individually motivated, self-initiated physical activity engagement.

Ain' Like There's Hunger

Sweet tooth
Salt tooth
Chocolate tooth
Jonesin' for fries,
Triple deck Mac,
Coke and pork rinds
But no walkin' tooth
Swimmin' tooth
Stretchin' tooth
Dancin' tooth
Weight liftin' tooth
After all,
Ain' like there's hunger . . .

Mind numbin' early gig
Second gig even worse
Kids in between
Gotta be fed
Read to
Homework checked
Ears inspected
Dark park?
Cold out?

After all,
Ain' like there's hunger . . .
Sittin' all day
Tryin' to look nice
'Do costin' thirty, fo'ty
Dollas a week
Heels and huggin' skirt
And these fifty extra pounds
I'm carryin' around
Stairs 're a joke!
Walkin' at lunch?
Humidity wreck my hair
After all,
Ain' like there's hunger . . .

TV and radio ads
For the Mickey Ds
KFCs
Taco Bells
Krispy Kremes
And Winchells
Seein' me, my kinda folks
Hearin' me, my kinda folks

It will require public and private sector involvement to craft a solution that gets people moving, soon and often. And in my view, critical private partners in selling this approach to organizations are marketing professionals. Not everyone can bring this expertise in-house, so the long-term collaborative arrangements that progressive state health departments have made with socially conscious marketing agencies, like Texas's EnviroMedia and California's Brown Miller Communications, are an excellent alternative model for developing this capacity. The other key partners are early adopter leaders who take the risk to disseminate innovations like *Instant Recess* in the workplace, persuaded of the value to their organizations' bottom lines.

"Ain' Like There's Hunger" is a poem I wrote some years ago to intro-

Golden arches
Right 'round the corner
Open late
Open early
Open twenty-fo/seven!
And then there's hunger . . .

CEOs
Makin' all this money
Makin' us fat and old
And sick and <u>dead</u>
Fat bankrolls
Phat money
"Blood" money
'S what it really is
Expandin' bottom lines
Expandin' our be-hinds
And waistlines
'Cause after all
Ain' like
There's real hunger!

So if bein' a nation
Of couch potatoes

Or "mouse" potatoes
Is really that bad
Why don't they
Make it easy?
Perk me up
Since I'm usually down
Where I work
On the "company's" clock

Yeah, how 'bout a little recess?
Like when we were
Kids in school
I might take a stroll
On "their" time!
Or find some jammin' tunes
For my little group
Packin' some extra pounds
Been a while since we got down!
"Shiftin' & movin' &
swingin' & groovin'"
Get that *natural high* flowin'
Now <u>that</u> might make me hungry
For more!

T___ *(June 23, 2003)*

duce a themed issue of the *American Journal of Preventive Medicine*—my first commissioned poem—created on demand!

SCIENCE, LIKE POLITICS, IS USUALLY PERSONAL

I know I've said several times that all the knowledge in the world about overeating and exercising won't motivate most folks to get healthy. It might be the same for me, but for a couple of really strong motivators to be active myself because of my family medical history—aside from vanity and a desire to hold on to my identity as an athlete. I'm sure that what I know, and especially what I've seen as a doc, make the threat to my own health and independence that much more real.

First, I'm on a crash course toward at least one knee replacement because of a hereditary, early onset, and rapidly progressive form of osteoarthritis that's ravaged the women in my family. I'm talking an average of two replacements apiece among my mom and her three sisters. The one that resisted (who I'm named after) ended up in a wheelchair by the time she died, albeit at age ninety. I'm on my first arthroscopy on my right knee and the third on my left. That one's got little remaining cartilage, and I want to be in the best shape possible when they put the new one in, so I can still play basketball and tennis after rehab.

The second and scariest, though, is that my mom and her next-older sister developed Alzheimer's in their mid- to late seventies, and we've got serious longevity genes. Granted, each of them had lost her husband of half a century a few years before the onset, on the heels of some major grieving and depression, and, as adults, they were much more sedentary than the two older sisters who were less traditional women, not coincidentally like me—childless (biologically, anyway) and headstrong and determined and adaptable and persistent and trailblazing. I hope, like them, I'm sharp practically till the day I leave the planet. But I don't have the same recall of my hundred most frequently called phone numbers and the near-photographic memory I used to. Hopefully, the former can be explained away by the crutch of my smart phone's touch dialing, and the latter can be chalked up to menopause.

She Went Away

Alzheimer's
Steals
Robs
Takes
Drains
Eradicates

Insidiously
Assiduously
Unrelentingly

A knowing smile
An arched eyebrow
A "stop you in your tracks" stare
A hearty laugh
A nervous glance
A sarcastic chuckle
A made-up word
Good glugallywogallywomblebot!

1% here
2% there
She
Slipped out
Seeped through
Was spirited away

Like sweat through her pores
Like tears through her eyelashes
Like blood from her veins
Like milk from her breasts
Like saliva from her lips

The memories
Of a life well lived
The pride
Of a life much appreciated
The confidence
Of a life much heralded
The dreams
Of a life lived vibrantly

The aspirations
Of a life well accomplished
The worries
Of a life lived responsibly

The entitlements
Of a life lived securely
The judgments
Of a life lived conventionally
The fears
Of a life lived cautiously
The concerns
Of a life lived conscientiously
The anxieties
Of a life lived squeamishly
The battles
Of a life lived defensively
The wounds
Of a life lived righteously

But not

The love
Of a life well connected
The *presence*
Of a life lived reverently
The hopes
Of a life well anchored
The satisfaction
Of a life lived appreciatively
The joys
Of a life lived simply
The contentedness
Of a life well protected
The gratitude
Of a life lived serenely
The graciousness
Of a life lived socially

Nor

(continued)

The frustrations
After a life lived independently
The timidity
After a life lived courageously
The prejudices
Of a life lived provincially
The resentments
Of a life lived collectively
The grudges
Of a live lived pettily
The aura
Of a life lived pretentiously

At what point
Has the *person*
Seeped out
Slipped through
The pores
The cracks
The holes
The fissures
The crevices
The quakes
The fault lines
The fractures
The cavities
The gaps
The interstices
The marks
The mucosa
The follicles
The sulci
The auricles
The marks
The retina
The pits
The grooves
The blemishes
The wounds

The cuts
The cuticles
The abrasions
The scars
The scrapes
The vacuum

At what point
Is the *person*
No longer there?
Behind the façade
Of the vacant stare
The hollow laugh
The angry countenance
The desperate clinging
The empty smile
The desolate look
The crumbling features
The reedy voice

A Hollywood set
Windows without sashes
Streets without gutters
Lawns without sprinklers
Chimneys without flues
Rain without clouds
Snow without frost
Grass without dew
Houses without foundations

When is a life
No longer worth living?
On some level
She knew
And she left
And she spared me
An Alzheimer's death.

                    T___· *(August 16, 2008)*

Unfortunately, I know from experience that Alzheimer's treatments are of modest utility at best, though Mom lived eleven years when the average time from diagnosis to death is seven years. She died of a sudden stroke or heart attack in her sleep and still recognized me most of the time until she passed away. Amazingly, she could read until the end, though that may not be so surprising in a woman with an under-grad degree in English and a master's degree in education who taught and tutored for more than sixty years. Her illness, nonetheless, was a decade-long agony in slow motion for my brother and me. Alzheimer's is the worst thing I could possibly wish on myself or my loved ones, and exercise and intellectual stimulation are currently the only known preventive measures. My job keeps the latter covered, and I doubt I'll ever completely retire. But my family history makes me want to stack the deck in my favor as much as possible. The poem I wrote at the time of Mom's passing may give you a sense of why preserving both my mobility and mental acuity mean that a day rarely goes by when I don't do something to contract some large muscles, breathe a little faster, and get my heart rate up.

FOUR

The Marketing and Social Marketing of
Physical Activity and Fitness

WHY A MARKETING PERSPECTIVE?

To get people to move, you have to seduce them a bit—sell them on
its attractiveness and immediate utility in their lives. And *immediate*
for most people rarely involves their health until catastrophe strikes
and they have a heart attack or stroke or cancer diagnosis. "Need an
energy boost?" "Want to be sexy?" If those appeals work for sports
drinks and push-up bras, they can work for physical activity—*if* the
costs and convenience are comparable. Big if! You really have to match
apples and apples. If the sports drink with the eye-catching label is in
the break room vending machine a stone's throw from your desk, or the
tantalizing aroma of coffee beckons from the reception area espresso
machine around the corner, but the walking path is on the other side of

the parking lot and there's nary a sign to remind you that it's there, or the barren stairs smell musty and are tucked away in the building interior, far from the entrance . . . those are obviously apples and oranges!

The cornerstone of health promotion, as I noted earlier, is making the healthy choice *easy* and the unhealthy choice increasingly difficult. This is how the battle against Big Tobacco has been waged successfully. Social marketing addresses socially beneficial behavioral change, behaviors that contribute to the public good individually and collectively. It offers a framework for understanding human desires and other drivers of behavioral change: how they compare with actual human needs and how to intervene effectively, in this case, to get people moving. Unlike commercial marketing, however, which aims to persuade people to purchase something whether or not they need it, social marketing sells a needed product, service, or idea (Grier and Bryant 2005). Social marketing borrows from commercial marketing its customer orientation and the four Ps, in hierarchical order: *product* (what is being offered—the benefit), *price* (what the consumer can exchange for the benefit), *place* (where services are provided, products distributed, or information received), and *promotion* (how services or products are offered). The customer represents a defined *population*, or target audience, and may be considered another P. The audience is rarely homogeneous, so audience segmentation is necessary to understand and reach different groups. There are also three tertiary Ps—*policy*, *partners*, and *politics*. I'll delve into these Ps in great detail later.

There is abysmally little commercial mass marketing for physical activity, as our study of outdoor advertising suggests (see chapter 2). Even targeted marketing of tennis rackets, tee times, stability balls, and personal trainers is limited to upscale venues and vehicles such as in-flight airline magazines, affluent neighborhoods, university alumni magazines, and TV shows catering to high-income demographics. Just think about televised golf and tennis tourneys. A lot more ads there for rackets, balls, and club memberships than during basketball and soccer games for balls, goals, and court or field rentals. Sedentary pursuits, on the other hand, are aggressively marketed, though nothing like the $33 billion annual tally that Big Food racks up (Institute of Medicine 2006). This leaves a definite niche for the mass marketing of physical activity.

EVOLUTION OF THE PUBLIC FACE OF
PHYSICAL ACTIVITY

In its earliest incarnation more than half a century ago, any exertion beyond work, chores, or travel was synonymous with exercising—either to "reduce" (the polite term for middle-aged portly women who were attempting to lose weight, not the current striving to look like a 13-year-old Barbie doll) or to enhance sex appeal. Exercises consisted of calisthenics to enhance the bust line, melt cellulite from cottage cheese thighs, or, in boys and men, build Charles Atlas biceps and pecs to escape embarrassment and bullying on the beach. Sales appeals for gimmicks, gadgets, and potions supporting these activities came in the ladies' magazine ads for vibrator belts, and pulp magazine ads for muscle stimulators, diet pills, and supplements aimed at teenagers and young adults. These entreaties were augmented by offerings from an embryonic stage of the now-booming fitness book industry. Just as is true today, these books were a mixed bag of sound advice, common sense, quackery, manipulation, and misrepresentation.

Early fitness icons, more embodiments of physical ideals of masculinity and femininity than pitch men and women, were generally established film stars and pinup models of the period, such as Johnny Weismuller and Jane Russell. Media representations of exercise and fitness subsequently diverged. The bodybuilding movement spun off as a sideshow, epitomized by the success of Lou Ferrigno and Arnold Schwarzenegger. In the meantime, Jack LaLanne, who mixed aerobic-type exercises, calisthenics, weight training, and good nutrition on his TV show, became the poster boy for the modern lifestyle gurus dominating the mainstream media.

The promotion of physical activity in the private sector through both nonprofit and commercial establishments has since been on the rise. Spa retreats and country clubs catering to the wealthy and elite have always maintained a background profile, the former in the tradition of the Western Health Reform Institute founded in the mid-1800s by the early Seventh Day Adventists and later transformed by John Harvey Kellogg into the Battle Creek Sanitarium. Private health clubs began to expand beyond social register clientele in the 1980s, when aerobics

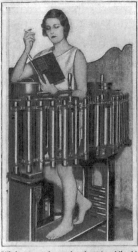

Beauty Machine Removes Excess Flesh Without Exercise

FASHION moguls have decreed that the boyish figure is passé, and that graceful curves are to be the coming mode. So, anticipating a need among the women, a far-sighted inventor has devised an instrument which literally rolls these curves into the body, getting rid of excess flesh without developing unsightly bundles of muscles, which exercising gave.

An important feature of the new device, however, is that developing these curves requires no work, for milady can become stylish in this new machine while reading a book, smoking a cigarette, or even gossiping. Hips, the chief point of attack, are reduced by means of rollers which massage the flesh, as illustrated in the accompanying photo.

Milady can smoke, read and gossip while this unique machine rolls off excess pounds of flesh around the hips, giving graceful curves, which fashion experts have decreed to be the coming mode. Massaging is performed by the rollers.

Modern Mechanix, August 1931

Figure 13. Promising results with little to no effort has always been a mainstay of fitness industry marketing.

became popular, and have continued into the present day. For-profit health clubs and YMCA-type gyms that were formerly considered the domain of older boys and men now include franchises marketed to specific segments of the population such as women, teens, older folks, and young children, spanning the range from Gold's Gym (young hipster fitness buffs) to Curves (overweight middle-aged women) to My Gym (preschoolers).

Aerobic equipment was generally introduced in health clubs—from treadmills, punching bags, jump ropes, and stationary bicycles to stair climbers, skiing simulators, steps, recumbent cycles, elliptical cross-trainers, and stability balls—and then mass marketed to individual users. Of course, the same snake oil salesmen from decades earlier, in modern guise, continue to prey on gullible marks with too-good-to-be-true offers. Lord knows how many stationary bikes are now clothes-drying racks in America's basements or dens, or more likely discarded in landfills.

Ironically, the commercial promotion of physical activity has recently begun to include the providers of sedentary entertainment. Video games such as Dance Dance Revolution, Sony Eye Toy, and the Wii Fit offer a more active option for recovering couch and mouse potatoes. Some proof of this mobilization of the sedentary may be seen in the spate of injuries specific to any exercise fad, especially among weekend warriors (Das 2009).

Health foundations actually played an active role in the development of physical gaming. Aggressive foundation support of the electronic gaming industry in developing physical or active video games represents a public-private partnership model that may have applications for recess breaks. This support came in the form of sponsoring interdisciplinary conferences, offering scholarships and awards, underwriting the development or expansion of university computer science gaming programs, and grant making to speed commercial application. These activities and opportunities raised the profile of physical gaming, attracting talented young scientists.

Key commonalities with the dissemination of activity breaks are the mutual benefit derived from the relationship central to the missions of each, the exploitation of new electronic information technologies, and the opportunities for rapid and mass diffusion. Several differences are also noteworthy. Active video gaming's emphasis is on individual and family participation, aside from some marketing to schools for use in physical education and to video arcades (such as with Dance Dance Revolution). The ability to try out active games is also somewhat limited because of the necessity for a relatively expensive upfront purchase, though this is offset to some extent by opportunities to sample the products at the homes of friends and extended family. Another challenge to electronic gaming is estimating demand and matching supply—the Nintendo Wii often sold out of retail outlets after its introduction, which may have suppressed sales and hampered dissemination.

Structured activity breaks, on the other hand, require little to no upfront investment, are unlimited in supply, encourage innovation especially by youth, and may be immediately acted upon after exposure to the promotional message. Last, the motivation for adoption of active gaming mostly operates at the individual level, as is true for the traditional paradigm for physical activity promotion. Gaming does drive motivation beyond individual enjoyment or health improvement to social interaction and reinforcement—fun, competition, and camaraderie. The motivation to incorporate activity breaks is vested in a leadership driven by existing incentives and disincentives for performance outcomes, visibility, or political expediency. But there have to be some sparks flying! Created by us sparkplugs: forward thinkers in physical activity and public health research and practice who can convince the involved stakeholders and decision makers of the utility of this approach.

The early social marketing of physical activity was done masterfully four decades ago by Ken Cooper. The prior public health focus on physical activity from the 1950s was on the increased risk of heart disease and premature death associated with long periods of occupational sitting, for example, among working-class bus drivers and mail sorters (Brown, Bauman, and Owen 2009). Dr. Cooper and his epidemiology chief, Steve Blair, were at the leading edge of the shift to a scientific focus on the benefits of activity in the form of structured leisure time exercise. Thus, the aerobics movement grew out of an affluent American white male sensibility and a medical versus public health perspective, which persists in physical activity promotion circles to this day. They spearheaded today's dominant paradigm, reflecting their cultural values and opportunities, namely, individualism, an inclination toward sports over dance, ample discretionary time and income, and a strong preference for thin women. Attention to culture is key, and that's why the aerobics movement was quite successful in its mass marketing efforts to mobilize these men— through mainstream media, the workplace (executive wellness is still the Cooper Institute's bread and butter), and other social institutions serving that demographic.

Women were left behind initially, because vigorous exercise and its sweating and panting and heavy weights and baggy workout clothing were incompatible—tacitly, if not explicitly—with the feminine socialization process. However, the commercial market represented by middle- and upper-class women, and the opening of sports opportunities to girls by the women's rights movement (Title IX), have spawned a burgeoning culture of physical activity participation. This has been spurred on and reinforced by tailored clothing and equipment proportioned for women's bodies (let's hear it for sports bras), group activity usually incorporating dance or music (aerobic dance, step, spinning, boxercise, and Pilates classes), and media representations of women exercising as normal. The early faces of this market, Jane Fonda and Brigitte Nielsen, have been succeeded by other exercise impresarios, including both men and women—Richard Simmons, Madonna, Billy Blanks, Oprah, and even Gwyneth Paltrow. Younger adult white women have pretty much caught up to men in activity levels, though this may be attributable, in part, to declining physical activity among males.

But those responding to these marketing appeals are still in the minority, and leisure time physical activity has never really penetrated the masses of adults in America, including less affluent communities and communities of color. The truth of this is reflected in their dismally low physical activity levels, despite the many low-cost or no-cost opportunities to engage in active recreation today. Most large corporations have on-site fitness facilities available for employee use before or after work, during lunchtime—or anytime, if you're an executive. City, county, and state governments, the largest employers in many locales, together with small and medium-sized private companies, consistently offer free or reduced-price memberships to health clubs with a broad geographic reach. For example, 24 Hour Fitness has partnered with NBA stars Magic Johnson and Shaquille O'Neal to establish high-quality gyms in low-income, ethnic minority neighborhoods that have never enjoyed such amenities and to thereby demonstrate their economic viability. Yet the main users of these fitness options are those who already regularly engage in activity on their own time and dime. The mere presence of active recreation facilities and spaces does not address the majority, or even the most important, of the barriers to physical activity participation; hence the need for intervention approaches informed by social marketing.

This pattern of leisure physical activity trends and fads remaining contained within the American elite may be continuing with the burgeoning green movement connection—devices and even clothing fibers that convert sweat equity into electrical power. The electricity may be channeled into a fuel cell and stored for other uses, or may directly supply a computer or other "screen" device in real time use by its human "generator." The proponents, marketing venues, communication vehicles, and pricing speak only to a select group—highly educated, Web savvy, and unlikely to derive meaningful benefits from either the energy expended or produced, given their propensity to exercise and ability to afford fuel of any type. Recently, however, these technological innovations have begun to seep into environmental applications, like the stairsteps with a little "give" in them such that each compression generates energy that can be stored—similar to solar panels or wind turbines. If employees were given monetary incentive give-backs based on the energy savings to the company, that might prove sufficient motivation to get them treading the stairwells in droves!

Promotion is the most visible component of social marketing, which feeds the misconception that social marketing relies primarily on advertising to achieve its aims. However, if an initiative stops there, it's merely the launch of a media campaign. For example, catchy ads were the primary nationwide investment by the feds in the Small Step campaign to encourage physical activity. Love handles and potbellies were mysteriously found on the beach, lost and abandoned after pudgy white guys took up walking. However, attention to place, product, and price is crucial to mounting an effective social marketing campaign. Which may have been a hurdle for the Small Step campaign in getting better traction. In contrast, JFK's fitness promotion initiative for schoolchildren translated the president's youth and popularity into rallying, monitoring, and incentives on the ground floor—at the school. This approach is resurfacing in a newer form, with advocacy groups using the Cooper Institute–derived FitnessGRAM as a source of data to apprise legislators, school officials, and parents of performance and progress, or the lack thereof.

WHY MARKETING? WHY NOW?

One of my greatest frustrations is the orthodoxy that emphasizing the benefits of brief bouts of exercise will erode the message advocating 30 minutes or more a day. First of all, the message isn't getting through, so there *is* no message. But the paradigm is also built on the flawed assumption that knowledge is both necessary and sufficient for behavioral change.

Some ivory tower types assert that contradictory recommendations from expert panels deter activity. The tiny population segment (self-selected volunteers) that attends to and values expert opinion is more affluent and active than most and quite adept at extracting and acting on salient information. For one thing, they're deathly afraid of getting old and gaining weight.

On the other hand, neither knowledge nor concern about health drives activity among the majority, as should be intuitively obvious from the dismal failure of all of this education to keep people active after research studies end or program funds run out . . . or even after the first few months of a study or program. So what happens? People drop out or fall off because they suddenly forget all that great information we taught 'em? The private sector provides a window, vis-à-vis fitness industry operations, on the behavior of people more advantaged and motivated to get active than the average person. Ask any health club manager or executive. Their business plan depends on selling the same workout space over and over again. According to the National Health Club Association, during the first year after joining, median "burnout" time for new members is three to four months, at which time approximately 50 percent discontinue regular attendance and payments. It is a misconception, perpetuated by aggressive health club advertising, that all or even most individuals joining gyms exercise at recommended levels. Most of those consistently attending are not meeting federal guidelines. Of the 50 percent attrition (those not completing their initial contract), 25 percent are inconsistent attenders and 25 percent are nonattenders. In subsequent years, loss rates (those completing the initial contract but not renewing) are 65–80 percent nationally, with "good" clubs averaging 40–55 percent. However, much depends on the club's organizational philosophy—for example, Bally's nearly exclusive focus on new recruitment. New sales necessitate attrition, or tremendous overcrowding of facilities would occur. This is supported by pilot data from our UCLA Fighting Cancer with Fitness study that got the great *LA Times* coverage. More than a third of the participants had been members of gyms or weight loss centers in the past.

On the Physical Activity Guidelines Advisory Committee that I mentioned earlier, several of us tried and failed to push beyond our charge to focus on the easy questions of how much, what, and why, in order to grapple with the more critical and less clear-cut questions of when, where, and how that would have made the best use of our think tank vetting process. The rollout of our report in October 2008 represented a critical missed opportunity to draw attention to the latter topics and to present a thoughtful digest of the best evidence available on the dissemination and implementation of physical activity interventions. The release apparently excited the public health community, as evidenced by the standing-room-only crowds when we presented the guidelines at professional meetings in the aftermath of the release. But the public health community splash barely registered as a blip on the mass media radar screen. I've yet to find anyone, outside of the field, even journalists covering health, who are even aware that there are new guidelines, much less what they are.

Of course, in all fairness, this lack of traction and visibility resulted as much from the timing and lack of controversy necessary to feed media interest, as from any flawed promotional strategy. There weren't many slow news days on the eve of electing the first African American president of the United States, as the country faced the worst economic slowdown since the Great Depression of the 1930s and monitored the mounting casualties of an increasingly unpopular war. The committee's admonitions to limit kids' computer and TV time and everyone's driving somehow failed to draw protests from lobbyists for the automobile, oil, highway construction, computer game, film, and TV industries . . . unlike the firestorm of protest by dairy, sugar, soda, cattlemen's beef, and fast food corporation lobbyists when the new dietary guidelines were released. Physical activity somehow just hasn't succeeded in getting people's attention. To be frank, we've not succeeded even in getting attention within the health field. Nowhere was this more apparent than in the Obama administration's health forums in 2009. In theory, health policy is broad, encompassing physical, cognitive, and emotional well-being. This makes sense, since only one-tenth of people's health status is influenced by what happens in hospitals and doctors' offices. In practice, however, health policy boils down to medical care policy. Fortunately, the National Physical Activity Plan Coordinating Committee has taken up where the Physical Activity Guidelines Advisory Committee left off, with a national launch in the works for May 2010 at the time of this writing.

Unfortunately, the rule and not the exception is that medical care sucks up all the air in the room, leaving public health gasping for breath, even though public health measures like widespread physical activity participation would improve the health of Americans and relieve a medical care system at the breaking point. We as a society just haven't grasped that we can't treat our way out of this health crisis, the lion's share of which is attributable to the epidemic of obesity and chronic disease. We simply don't have the time, political will, system capacity, or money—and the latter should be of prime concern in a serious recession. We're going to have to dam the flood upstream, not just bail the water downstream.

So we've got a lot of behavior to change en route to becoming an active nation, and the behavior of key decision makers is a central part of that journey. There are several ways to influence voluntary behavioral change: education and communication, marketing, policy, and legal advocacy, or some combination of these. *Education and communication* involve activities that change the information environment for the purpose of informing people or organizations about options they currently have. Education and communication change knowledge, but simply knowing doesn't equate to doing. *Marketing* refers to activities that change the competitive market environment for the purpose of providing people or organizations with new options that are intended to be more attractive than their current options. *Policy and legal advocacy* encompass activities that change—or are intended to change—regulations and laws for the purpose of providing incentives for or mandating certain options, or providing disincentives for or prohibiting other options. Of course, if you're a member of Congress, a city council, or a state senate, you can skip the advocacy (except among other members) and directly set policy.

When should we use each option? According to physical activity market research genius Ed Maibach, there are several key factors to consider. You have to gauge how strongly people are inclined to behave as desired, how readily the benefits can be conveyed, and what the level of competition is. Education and communication work fine if people are prone to behave as desired, if self-interest or benefits are easy to convey, and if there's little or weak competition. Marketing can be employed when people are neither prone nor resistant to the behavior promoted, when self-interest can be conveyed by pumping up the offer (through incentives like free samples or short-term discounts to get them started and hopefully reaping intrinsic benefits like cost savings, and feeling or looking better), and when there's active competition. Changes in policies and laws are the last recourse, when people are resistant to adopting the behavior, self-interest can't be conveyed easily, and the competition is unmanageable.

Of course, it's something of a mixed bag. Competition comes from within and without in the case of physical activity. As I've discussed, people are resistant to the desired behavior by nature—genetic programming that was adaptive for most of the time we've been on the planet. And the outside competition is fierce, probably unmanageable—cars, screens, gaming, and PDAs (they're called CrackBerrys for a reason). Self-interest *can* be conveyed by enhancing the offer (what people get for their time and money or sweat), but that has yet to be done in a way that moves the masses of adults: targeting the offers to organizations rather than individuals, and exploiting the organizational infrastructure—social networks, communications, performance measures, the physical plant, market competition, leader competitiveness, culture, and values.

WHAT WE DID, AND WHY AND HOW WE DID IT

I've talked about what social marketing is and when it's used. So the question now is how to get it done. The following are examples of various elements of my teams' marketing of physical activity within several projects I directed in Los Angeles and in Richmond, Virginia, including sample materials and messages. They illustrate each of the classic four Ps of marketing and a few more. This history pointed the way to the present. As you'll see, cultural resonance is a consistent theme.

Fighting Cancer with Fitness: Promotion and Place

As an African American cultural insider researcher, I understood that feelings of exploitation and exclusion, but also community spirit, shared destiny, and pride in the accomplishments of those overcoming the odds are common themes in African American culture, so study recruitment materials were designed to tap into these attitudes and emotions. Colorful postcards and fliers asserted, "When programs are developed to fight cancer and heart disease, our voices must be heard. After all, our tax dollars are paying for it." The letter of introduction began, "Dear Sister . . . " and noted that the gym study site was black owned and operated, and the principal investigator (me) was an African American physician (Yancey et al. 2001).

However, a message can work only if it reaches the target audience. My MBA guru Octavia Miles suggested that we purchase blocks of names of subscribers to *Essence*, the health and beauty magazine for African American women, living within a ten-mile radius of the health club study site; and we got great coverage in the *LA Times*. But our greater-than-anticipated recruitment success came through social networks. Three-quarters of the participants heard of the study from a personal contact. Obese women were particularly likely to come to us through word of mouth—we inferred that heavier women needed reassurance that this opportunity was appropriate for them, not for the buffed babes and muscle-bound men in the Bally's ads. Place came into play here, because the location and parking were central and convenient. The gym itself was also different from our prospective participants' stereotypes. Not only was it populated by older, heavier folks than the models in fitness club ads, but it also featured décor chosen to appeal to women, and some machines sized shorter for the average woman. This project highlights many elements of the concept of *promotion*, or how services or products are offered, via messaging, framing, messengers, and channels. These activities include audience test marketing, advertising, public relations, and on-site purchase incentives like prompts, coupons, and product samples. This is only the tip of the iceberg, so to speak, but if it's not done well, you can have a great product in the perfect place at the right price, and it still won't sell.

It helps if the framing is creative and catchy. I usually get a collective "Hmmm . . . hadn't quite looked at it that way" when I say that I can deliver the equivalent of one-third of the recommended daily allowance (RDA) for physical activity in the form of a 10-minute exercise break, a lot more cheaply and easily than I can a nutrient-rich meal. I get a similar response, perhaps laced with a dose of healthy skepticism, when I communicate my vision that people come to feel the same sense of entitlement to exercise breaks as they do to coffee breaks. But, even better, my colleague Dr. Bill Releford gets hoots and hollers when he calls dollar-menu fast-food burgers "99-cent weapons of mass destruction!"

Proper framing is crucial because it changes the perceived value of a good or service and thereby enhances the benefit that offsets the price or cost of the behavioral change. It can be as important to avoid a negative connotation as to emphasize the positive. For example, when I took over Fitness Fanatics, the state-funded physical activity promotion program at Charles R. Drew University, we kicked around the idea of changing the project's name during our early community advisory committee meetings. It turned out that most committee members did not like the original idea of labeling participants as fitness fanatics. That seemed to fit neither the reality nor the goal. We wanted to get a lot of folks to move around a bit, preferably without even seeing it as exercise, not drum up fanaticism for fitness among a few. We also toyed with Fitness Fun-addicts, but people were very clear that "we don't need anybody addicted to anything else down here in South Central LA!" So someone came up with Fitness *Fun*atics, and that name stuck—it was consistent with our framing of activity as enjoyable and enthusiastically embraced by the staff and participants for the duration of the project.

Social math is an example of a framing approach. It's about trying to come up with a way to communicate statistics that resonates with people—regular folks and health professionals. I was on an obesity seminar panel with Jay Olshansky a few years after he published his projection that members of this generation may be the first to live shorter lives than their parents since the government started keeping mortality stats. He said that he'd planned to submit the article to another journal, and just serendipitously, happened to mention the study to a *New England Journal of Medicine* editor. This compelling statistic got him into the premier medical journal, and a "shot heard round the world" avalanche of citations and coverage in the medical and lay media.

Another framing strategy is positioning a health behavior as the antithesis of its popular image. My recess model is predicated on framing physical activity as fun versus work, summoning images of freedom and whimsey versus joyless, slavish, perfunctory "pulling teeth." It's not only shifting from a negative to a positive image, but the contrast may also be attention getting. A parallel may be seen in smoking-cessation or HIV-prevention public service announcements shifting from invoking a fear of disease to enhancing one's sex appeal by not smoking (fewer facial wrinkles, better smelling breath and clothes) and to enhancing sexual pleasure and novelty with colorful and flavorful condoms, and showing sexy models using them, thereby making condom use sexy.

The "recess" label also reframes the opportunity for physical activity during the workday as an entitlement. This could help in getting unions on board to prevent their members from being *deprived* of movement necessary to their physical and mental well-being or to demand its inclusion in preventive health care benefits packages, tapping into the loss aversion that's part of human nature (see chapter 3). This, again, is the polar opposite of many adults' feelings of being forced to exercise as children—being made to participate in sports by a gung-ho parent or having to run laps as punishment for inadequate performance by drill instructor coaches or PE teachers. Finally, physical activity may be presented as a worker injury *given*—an obvious and necessary safety precaution that employers would be remiss or even exploitive or legally liable in omitting. This stance is wonderfully illustrated by L. L. Bean's wellness coordinator, who characterized the company's mandatory 5-minute stretch breaks as a safety measure—like requiring safety glasses (Simon 2006).

This view of physical activity as an occupational safety measure stands in stark contrast to a prevailing and misguided employer concern about *increased* liability exposure from employees engaging in physical activity at work—to the point that some even discourage stair use to avoid workers' compensation claims. Maybe people wouldn't injure themselves during such mundane activities if they weren't cooped up for hours at a time, often in close quarters, like chickens in a henhouse!

Prolonged sitting and repetitive motion is certainly much more hazardous to the health than moderate activity. Inactivity interferes with cognitive processing, impairs cardiovascular functioning, dampens mood, atrophies muscles, depletes bone mass, and robs tendons and ligaments of their tone and flexibility.

Teen Activity Project (TAP): Product and Price

We received funding for TAP, which targeted teen girls, from a program funded by the settlement of a class action suit against General Foods for the predatory marketing of sugary cereals to preschool African American and Latino children. By the time the monies came, the children affected were mostly tweens (nine to thirteen years old). This was my first foray into incorporating dance into a public health effort. A practical lesson subsequently emerged. Since the teens leading the classes were talented dancers, often cheerleaders for the school's sports teams, the routines quickly became complex and aerobically taxing, leaving the less fit and coordinated girls in the dust. In addition, the fear of disturbing hair and makeup was front and center as a deterrent to being active (Taylor et al. 1999). Less vigorous and rigorous movements adapted for the rhythmically or aerobically challenged were the order of the day (Leslie et al. 1999). Clearly, if we were to get the least active folks moving comfortably and enjoyably, we had to keep it simple and modest in intensity.

TAP offers a prime example of the importance of the *product*, or what is being offered: that is, the benefit. The benefit must be perceived to be a more attractive option than the current behavior, or the consumer won't make the exchange. For behavioral changes such as increasing physical activity that may incur some discomfort (perceived exertion, feelings of inadequacy, muscle soreness, sweatiness) and that result in mostly delayed benefits, incentives such as sporting goods store gift cards and pedometers may be key in sweetening the deal. They may help tremendously in the adoption and habituation. However, establishing monitoring and evaluation mechanisms for providing feedback and highlighting and documenting short- and longer-term benefits are important for sustainability. This is particularly relevant for organizational-level outcomes, such as productivity improvements or decreased leave, in order to encourage the continuation or expansion of policies permitting physical activity on paid work time and, ultimately, the institutionalization of such policies.

One aspect of TAP addressed a variation of *price*, in this case, the cost of engaging in the behavior promoted. The price is what the customer *must* exchange, usually time, money, or both. So the price must be right—if it's too high, the customer will either stay put or seek alternative options. A product that can be used without great inconvenience to the participant costs less. In TAP, simple moves averted the costs of embarrassment, and modest intensity reduced the costs to girls of disturbing their hair and makeup.

Fuel Up/Lift Off! LA/¡Sabor y Energía!: *Promotion, Place, and Price*

Fuel Up/Lift Off! LA (the Spanish-language literal interpretation is something like "Sizzle" or "Gusto and Energy") was a Los Angeles County Department of Public Health social marketing campaign promoting recess breaks in organizations, funded by the state health department and the USDA. The idea was to make physical activity—in bite-sized doses—and nutrient-rich food choices accessible, appealing, and just part of the normal way of doing business. We tested the campaign by providing six weekly 30-minute on-site training sessions followed by three on-site booster sessions during the subsequent year, delivered by county health educators. By the third session, a "program champion" (Wellness Warrior) from within the organization was identified and empowered by the site leadership and county project staff to assist in sustaining behavioral and organizational changes after the initial training period, to serve as a conduit for project materials and communications, and to represent the organization at quarterly training seminars conducted at county offices. We recruited two sites with 15 people for a pretest, and then tested *Fuel Up/Lift Off!* in seven sites with 114 people. Preliminary three-month pretest-posttest follow-up results revealed some positive changes, including an increase in weekly strength or toning exercises, and possibly fewer people that were totally sedentary (Yancey, McCarthy, et al. 2006). However, the evaluation was discontinued prematurely due to county funding cuts the next year, although the campaign continued to recruit organizations and train their staffs.

Framed positively around the benefits of healthy eating and active living, rather than negatively around obesity control, the project was modeled on commercial ad campaigns targeting African American and Latino communities with images conveying energy, enjoyment, excitement, and social interaction, similar to campaigns for products like beer and soda. Since my creative director, Todd, used to design such ads for Miller Beer and McDonald's, we had a head start.

We felt it important to emphasize physical activity and de-emphasize weight loss in our messages because Los Angeles is the most culturally diverse metropolis in the nation, and there are vastly different cultural definitions of size and beauty. Getting people to label themselves as overweight may be unsuccessful if a person is considered small in her or his social circle. It's all relative. It may even be counterproductive: one of our studies demonstrated that non-obese people who thought they were overweight were *less* likely to be physically active, regardless of how much they weighed. Not to mention that people in some ethnic minority communities feel further stigmatized because their physical attributes do not and will never match the mainstream ideal. I often hear this from otherwise average-weight African Americans carrying some extra "junk in the trunk." This suggests that we probably do better when we feel better, not worse, about ourselves. Anecdotally, I hear a lot of people that say that having shed a few pounds gets them out the door to the gym faster than having gained a few—the latter more often sinking them further into their couches with ice cream or chips. This ties in with the price-lowering aspect: the promotion enhances the offer (highlighting salient, desirable, and elusive outcomes), while the convenience resulting from the captive-audience strategy (place) and perhaps compensation (for example, if exercise breaks or walking meetings occur on paid company time) lowers the cost of participation (price).

Using the Ps I talked about earlier, the organizationally based *Fuel Up/Lift Off!* speaks to *place*—where services are provided, products are distributed, or information is received. This is the real coup for a "captive audience" strategy like recess breaks. Not only do people *not* have to travel to participate, because they're already at work, but they are repeatedly exposed at work to prompts for the activity and the activity itself, as well as the social interactions surrounding the activity and cultural changes supporting the activity. People tend to think that marketing influences individuals, but people don't operate in isolation. On the contrary, much of the marketing influence on behavior is leveraged through social networks. Opportunities for social exchange and influence are enhanced by fairly uniform and ubiquitous exposure, in terms of the timing and number of contacts. This represents another mechanism by which people internalize behaviors formerly requiring extrinsic motivation—audiences whose admiration is sought and whose opinions matter (peers, colleagues, relatives, and so on) can strongly motivate adherence on an ongoing basis.

Fuel Up/Lift Off! also speaks to *price*, that is, what the consumer can exchange for the benefit. For blue- or pink-collar workers or administrative support staff punching a time clock, trading 10 minutes of dancing for 10 minutes of work may be an attractive alternative. That's less the case for upper-echelon salaried professionals who are held responsible, not for the time they spend at work, but rather for a certain volume of work or the results of that work, but that's OK. We're designing strategies that favor the more sedentary, higher-risk groups.

There are several tertiary Ps and a few newer marketing Ps: *partners* (alliances and coalitions with common goals); *politics, policies*, and powerful *players* that influence public climate and acceptability; and *purse strings*. Partners have often greased the skids and saved the day for me. The Association of Black Women Physicians in Los Angeles referred women to Fighting Cancer with Fitness, gave guest lectures, and put their political heft behind some enabling policies I supported. In Richmond, politics were on our side. The mayor's wife was a strong advocate, and other politicians were inclined to help because I'd promptly addressed a mosquito infestation in the district of one of the City Council members.

The flatline response to the release of the Physical Activity Guidelines for Americans illustrated the influence of another P—the *public climate*, the many outside factors that can make or break a marketing campaign.

The current US Department of Agriculture–funded campaign for healthy eating and physical activity, targeting people who use food stamps, provides an excellent example of purse strings—as in who controls the dollars. Very little of the money can be directed to physical activity because the origin of the funds places the focus squarely on nutrition, with the role of physical activity relegated to energy balance; physical activity can be demonstrated to people only a few times—funds cannot be used for the ongoing provision of exercise instruction; and the Bush administration precluded using funds for the broader social marketing efforts that were the original focus of the initiative rather than for the direct education of food stamp clients. In my opinion, the feds' motivation reflected Big Food's operating through bureaucrats to preclude advocacy for systems change. At least as much as anything else. The *anything else* being the public health establishment's underappreciation of, and underinvestment in, physical activity. Fortunately, the Obama administration is in the process of removing these restrictions and permitting states more latitude in marketing healthy eating and active living—with the trade-off that program expenditures are capped at current levels.

CURRENT ACTIVITY MARKETING CAMPAIGNS

There are a couple of recent examples of really well-done physical activity mass marketing campaigns. Not coincidentally, in both instances, the private sector played a central role, with public health driving the content and commercial marketing driving the dissemination. Each did what it does best.

Public Social Marketing: VERB—It's What You Do!

VERB was the brainchild of the Centers for Disease Control and Prevention, a chance to do it right, and the campaign developers took a lot of heat for the substantial level of funding, for once sufficient to get the job done. In VERB, tweens (nine- to thirteen-year-old pre- and early adolescents) were encouraged to participate in physical activity by choosing a verb such as *run, bike, dance, skate* as a starting point. A TV ad message was "Everywhere you go, everywhere you look, there are verbs out there just waiting for you to get into . . . "

The VERB campaign vividly demonstrated that culture counts. It ignored the disdain of adult public health academicians and practitioners and grounded its campaign messages in hip-hop culture. A huge budget by public health standards—in excess of $150 million by a direct congressional appropriation—was invested, mostly in engaging a top advertising firm.* The organizers tried hard to tie the campaign to ongoing youth group activities, as well as to state and local health department initiatives and parks and recreation programs that provided active leisure opportunities. In contrast to most public health interventions, the effects were initially greatest among ethnic minority populations, African American girls in particular (Huhman, Heitzler, and Wong 2004).

Private Marketing and Community Benefit: Kaiser Permanente's Thrive

The Thrive campaign, aimed at getting people to live healthier and happier lives and, not incidentally, differentiating the company from its competitors by making Kaiser seem warm and fuzzy, complements its Healthy Eating Active Living (HEAL) Initiative funded in part by its Community Benefit program.

Kaiser Permanente (KP) is the largest private, not-for-profit health care organization in the United States, with 8.6 million members, or beneficiaries. KP operates 35 medical centers, more than 430 medical offices, and a network of research units in nine states and the District of Columbia. The organization has 167,000 employees, 14,600 physicians practicing exclusively at KP, and annual revenues in excess of $40 billion.

HEAL promotes physical activity through:

---

*Unfortunately, as soon as brand visibility was achieved and successful outcomes demonstrated, the campaign was sacrificed to make room for President George W. Bush's tax cuts.

Delivery-system interventions. Evidence-based clinical-practice changes support the prevention and treatment of overweight, for instance, by training docs to write exercise prescriptions.

Community health initiatives. KP convenes schools, health departments, community organizations, and health care providers to develop strategies to change institutional practices, public policy, and the built environment.

Organizational practice changes. Health care organizations model wellness practices by increasing access to physical activity opportunities through on-campus walking trails and connections to public transit and other alternatives to driving, and by creating incentives for employees to exercise.

Public policy advocacy. KP funds advocacy organizations and backs legislation designed to make it easier for people to be active.

Advertising campaign. The Thrive ad campaign communicates KP's philosophy of prevention and health promotion and influences social norms with radio, TV, outdoor, and online spots. Colorful and fast-moving images against varied backdrops of energetic and upbeat people of both genders and varying ages, sizes, classes, and ethnicities dancing and playing, with mouthwatering shots of fruits and vegetables, convey KP's commitment to helping everyone "thrive." The few clinical settings depicted have been of happy doctors and healthy patients getting routine physicals, with death and disease nowhere in sight!

In 2009, KP was awarded the Centers for Disease Control and Prevention Pioneering Innovation Award, presented at the inaugural Weight of the Nation conference, for the Thrive campaign's influence on social norms about food and physical activity, combined with KP's work on the ground to change food and physical activity environments.

LOOKING TO THE FUTURE: A MODEL FOR THE SOCIAL MARKETING OF *INSTANT RECESS*

Given that California is the pioneer, innovator, and leader in population approaches to obesity and chronic disease prevention and control, the state could be poised to create the next national physical activity social marketing success. The same agency that developed the 5 a Day promotion for fruit and vegetable consumption, the California Department of Health Services (Foerster et al. 1995), now the Department of Public Health, supported the development of *Instant Recess* and its *Lift Off!* predecessor. Although it may seem like I'm comparing apples to oranges—or rather apples to modified jumping jacks—bear with me. The parallels between the evolution of 5 a Day and the emergence of *Instant Recess* are striking. Recess breaks could be seen as a comparable promotional message for physical activity to 5 a Day for fruit and vegetable intake. Like 5 a Day, *Instant Recess* conveys a simple, easily recalled and understood, and immediately doable action. Each of the two products may be attractively packaged. Also like 5 a Day, the recess message is consistent with the incremental nature of behavioral change. Adding 10 minutes to the typical US adult's 6 to 10 minutes a day of moderate to vigorous activity is within reach, in the same way that adding a serving or two to the average adult's three or four per day is not a huge leap.

Instant Recess may actually have a few advantages over 5 a Day, in that the product is cheaper and perhaps even as profitable as the competition (sedentary behavior-promoting products and services, such as traditional video games), the competition is not mobilized in opposition, and its success is aligned with the goals of several deep-pocket private industries. As people become more active, the market for sporting goods and equipment, fitness apparel, health club memberships, field and court rentals, and personal training will increase. This may also create more of an appetite for spectator sports and its collateral product sales. (As we've seen, teens who watch sports, for example, also play more sports than nonspectators.) Filling the coffers of professional sports franchises already predisposed to invest in physical activity promotion would increase their return on investment and ultimately their continued or expanded investment. Recess breaks do not present the problem of maldistribution from a public equity standpoint. They may be done anywhere, anytime, in any attire. The delivery mechanism (CD or DVD) may be distributed at minimal, if any, cost and reused (for example, it can be made available for streaming or downloading from the Internet). Fruits and vegetables are perishable with a short shelf life and low profit margin and consequently are much more readily purchased in affluent than poor neighborhoods. Recess breaks may be more readily picked up and disseminated by the private sector—the profit margin is there and existing distribution networks (traditional and virtual bookstores, DVD rental businesses, fitness industry retailers, wellness contractors) may be exploited.

There could be a few bumps in the road. The main disadvantage of *Instant Recess* compared with 5 a Day is that it flies in the face of physical activity promotion orthodoxy—it focuses on socially obligatory group activity (versus individually motivated solo activity) in amounts that don't meet the federal recommendations. Some power brokers of the scientific bureaucracy have been adamant that a public focus on the recess message undermines the chances of achieving regular physical activity as a nation because it implies that bouts of less than 30 minutes per day are sufficient. This is mind boggling to me (and others form- ing the minority opinion of the Physical Activity Guidelines Advisory Committee, as I mentioned earlier), since the segment of the population achieving the 30-minute recommendation is such a minority and so much less attuned to health news "sound bites" than the general public.

Susan Tufts, a twenty-year veteran of exercise-break implementation at the apparel and equipment retailer L. L. Bean, whom I interviewed for this book, strongly agreed that a more modest recommendation would be empowering for people who aren't meeting the guidelines. She indi- cated, in no uncertain terms, that in her experience, people tune out the 30-minute message as daunting and unattainable. She also said she'd often seen employees start small and build up almost automatically, as a natural progression accompanying physiological conditioning. And they're mostly blue-collar white guys where she works in Maine, a large and largely overlooked overweight and inactive population segment. Maybe they're understudied and underserved from the standpoint of physical activity promotion because people assume these guys get lots of exercise as construction workers, mechanics, and longshoremen. But those jobs have become scarce, much more mechanized, and much less strenuous, like the rest of the jobs in society—requiring a lot more fine- motor finger movement than large-muscle contraction and body motion.

The Real Gatekeepers

I know one group of people who could seriously make it happen, and whose role in health promotion has been grossly underappreciated, namely, journalists. Everybody's on board with working to understand the culture of the target population, and public health people are starting to zero in on the cultures of business and politics to understand what drives the decisions of these gatekeepers and influencers. But only a few public health investigators—Matt Kreuter at Washington University in St. Louis being a notable exception—and even fewer public health practitioners are talking about journalists and their culture—motivation, drivers, constraints, and the like.

So I'm throwing in my lot with the journalists! Shari Roan and that '94 *Los Angeles Times* article about our pilot study taught me a thing or two about reach and exposure, about what makes something memorable, and about what cuts through the crowded, sometimes oppressive information environment and seems fresh and inviting and motivating and inspiring.

I've benefited tremendously from their creativity over the years. For example, Gordon Hickey, a writer for the *Richmond Times Dispatch* who covered local government when I was there, was an alum of the venerable Iowa Writers' Workshop. Could he ever turn a phrase! The excerpt below is from his July 14, 1996, article introducing me to the city, titled "Dressing, Dribbling and Now Directing." In one fell swoop, Gordon's flattering portrayal conveyed a ringing endorsement from a very popular and high-profile city manager, laid out my agenda for my tenure there, burnished my academic credentials for Richmond's white elite, communicated my values and perspective and grounded them in black culture, linked me to a sports phenom in a place where high school football matters, touted my deep family ties to the region, and most critically, distanced me from California. The city manager and the police chief had also been recruited from California, which many non-Northern Virginians view as one step up from the seventh ring of hell—in no small part because they feel people in the Northeast and on the West Coast look down on them as hicks and underestimate their intelligence. (Gordon also wrote the "Richmond Mayor Rocks World of Physical Fitness" article shown in fig. 10 in the previous chapter.)

Antronette K. Yancey is a mile-a-minute rhyming dynamo with a medical degree and a mean jump shot.

She's a 6-foot-3-inch former basketball player, former international model, current physician and current writer who's coming to Richmond to be director of the city's Department of Health. . . .

Yancey "possesses outstanding qualifications as well as the enormous energy, enthusiasm and vision necessary for success," Bobb said. . . .

Yancey, 38, starts . . . officially on September 1. But she was in town recently to accept the position, buy a house and get the lay of the land.

During an interview in City Hall, she said she likes what she's found.

"I have roots here," she said. Though she was born and raised in Kansas City, Kan., her father was reared in Louisa County. Her 80-year-old aunt, Rebecca Thurston, still lives on the property there. . . .

"A number of things have happened that sort of directed me to Richmond," she said. Not the least of which is her 6-foot-5-inch godson who will attend Fork Union Military Academy. . . .

And then there's her poetry. She uses it in lectures on health issues to get across the emotion of her views. The poetry, dealing with issues such as desegregation, responsibility, sports and health, will be published soon in a collection called "An Old Soul with a Young Spirit." One poem called "The Village" goes this way:

This is a tribute
To all the brothas out there
My brothas
Our brothas
Raisin' they kids
Like they s'posed to
Like the gov'ment
Didn't want 'em to . . .

Yancey is a stylish eruption of ideas and visions. She is a display of rings, ear ornaments, bracelets and pins as she expounds on the village she wants to join here . . .

. . . about 70 percent of the problems that send patients to doctors are better dealt with by changes in behavior than by administering medications.

That means the Health Department will work with other agencies such as the Department of Parks and Recreation and the Police Department to make people healthier, Yancey said.

She also said she intends to use her talents to take her message of health, fitness, and general well-being to the streets. "Get it on the radio, get it on TV, make music videos. You have to take it to the people.". . .

One day last week, she walked from her downtown hotel up Church Hill. Along the way, she came up with an acronym for a program she wants to start in Richmond—SECEDE.

It stands for Self-Esteem through Creative Expression Defying Expectations. "I want to secede from the union of pain and suffering," she said.

She sees that happening through athletics and activity in general. "It allows [people] to get rid of negative emotions in a positive way," she said.

A couple of years later, when our coffee table poetry and art book came out (*An Old Soul with a Young Spirit: Poetry in the Era of Desegregation Recovery*), I really experienced firsthand the power of the media. A journalist friend got me an interview with the New York City Pacifica radio station, WBAI. I read several poems on air a few hours before I was a scheduled guest at my friend Harold James's regular poetry reading at a Lower East Side spot, the Telephone Bar and Grill. The back room only had about 50 seats, and by the time I performed, it was packed— standing room only. People were literally banging on the closed door and begging to at least be allowed to buy a book if they couldn't get in.

And LA-based NPR staff writer Patti Neighmond did a great segment on *Instant Recess* that aired in February 2009. The piece was followed by a Web-based dialogue hosted by NPR health editor Joe Neel on the "micro-exercise" movement (first time I ever heard that label) that attracted more than 400 people and had me typing as fast as I could for 45 minutes. They surveyed the people who tuned in, and 29 percent indicated that their employers already provided short exercise breaks— another 37 percent responded "I wish!" The story and blog are still on the NPR Web site along with Neighmond's Web-only synthesis of the lessons informing *Instant Recess* that's the best I've seen:

Exercising with a Crowd Is Easier

Yancey describes the mini-fitness sessions as a part of a "captive audience strategy." It can be tough to get some people to break their work routine even for 10 minutes to exercise, she says, though they'll have fun if they do. So sometimes, while addressing a conference, she will stop midway and tell the gathered crowd that they are going to stop for a little exercise. "People kind of frown, look around nervously, particularly those who are overweight or obese and not used to exercising in public," she says.

But once Yancey puts on the DVD and turns on the music, "they do it because everyone else is doing it." That's the key, she says. "We're social beings. The motivation is social." And, often, even short exercise breaks will entice people to adopt healthier lifestyles—better diets and exercise—over the long run.

Company Support Is Crucial

To make daily exercise a priority, top-down leadership is necessary for bottom-up support, Yancey says. Some companies have started pushing back from the conference table to institute "walking meetings" or even replaced the seats around the conference table with elliptical machines. As a start, she says, companies might institute a sort of "sitting" ban similar to smoking bans—at least during some meetings, for those who are able. The most successful intervention, she says, may require the CEO and other managers to join in a five- or 10-minute recess break like the sessions she teaches: a brief, low-impact, simple and structured group physical activity, usually done to music and integrated into the organizational routine at work.

The People Who Need It Most Will Get the Most Out of It

Critics sometimes squeal that short breaks don't raise the heart rate enough to help folks who are already in good shape lose weight or increase their fitness. That may be true. But they'll be refreshed and have fun, and it's the best way to get to others who are true couch potatoes. Yancey's studies show that even a little exercise in the afternoon increases the likelihood that people will take the extra initiative and get more exercise in the evening or on the weekend.

What's Good for the Worker Is Good for the Company

Retailer L.L. Bean instituted daily, mini-exercise breaks 15 years ago throughout its assembly plant with great results, Yancey says. The breaks were five minutes each, three times a day. At the end of the shift, the company found a 30-minute return on productivity for an investment of 15 minutes of physical activity. "The number of bags and shoes that they do not produce in those 15 minutes," she says, "they actually get back and then some." Yancey is now involved in a study looking at how employees fare at more than 70 work sites instituting similar programs across Los Angeles County. She expects findings within three years. (Neighmond 2009)

I also recruited John Rabe, a show host on the largest of the Southern California NPR affiliates, KPCC, and for whom I'd done public health commentaries for a couple of years, to help edit this book for lay audiences. Basically, I got him to retrain me to write the way I used to before getting on the tenure track and scientific "publish or perish" merry-go-round. Rabe must have done a good job: near the end of the project, after working with me to refine the message for inactive people like him sliding toward unhealthiness, he started riding his bike to work two or three times a week. (I can't swear to it, but I think his editing got better after he started getting more active.)

Most recently, having just attended one of my first meetings after I was appointed to the board of directors of the Partnership for a Healthier America (the nonprofit organization supporting first lady Michelle Obama's Let's Move initiative), I was tickled by an e-mail from Mona AuYoung, one of my doctoral students, with the subject line, "someone's in the news." A Reuters writer had penned an online story with the headline, "Routine Recess a Hit at White House Obesity Summit: A Doctor's Endorsement of Frequent Recess Breaks—and Not Just for Kids—Drew an Appreciative Response from Experts Meeting at a White House Summit on Childhood Obesity on Friday."

Instant Recess could be deemed a clear and present opportunity for California to maintain its front-runner status in disease prevention and health promotion established by tobacco control and 5 a Day. And the court of public opinion may gradually weigh in and drown out the skeptics, especially with the state's finances tanking and politicians scrambling to be seen as doing something constructive without spending any money.

THE MESSENGER AND THE MEDIUM

Marketing tries to reach or penetrate a target audience with a message that is effective in inducing a behavioral change. That change must be amplified or adopted widely, fully implemented, and maintained and sustained over a sufficient period of time to create lasting change in sociocultural norms, practices, and policies.

The most important aspect of that message is its resonance with the target audience and the credibility of its messenger for the product or service marketed. Marketing people refer to the latter as *homophily*—the degree of similarity between messenger and audience. For example, the TV show *ER*, in consultation with University of Southern California's Hollywood, Health & Society project, created a multi-episode storyline around a young, overweight black male character recurring over several episodes who regularly consumed fast food and ended up in the intensive care unit with congestive heart failure. Recall of those *ER* episodes in a subsequent opinion poll was significantly more likely to result in some evidence of behavioral change among African Americans and among men, like self-reported increases in fruit and veggie intake and walking a few blocks, than among other demographic groups (Valente et al. 2007). Those demographic segments, notoriously difficult to engage in health promotion efforts, would have been unlikely to attend to real doctors, patients, and hospitals, even if they had appeared in ads or public service announcements during the same popular show. Interestingly, exposure to this *ER* storyline among African Americans was not associated with greater knowledge or more favorable attitudes toward physical activity compared with those not exposed. With this lesson in mind, as you'll see in the next chapter, I've partnered with the Professional Athletes Council to promote the recess model. We're concentrating on the settings in which athletes have the greatest sway or leverage, namely sports venues and schools or other youth-serving programs. Athletes are often used as messengers in promoting fitness, and in our case, appropriately so for the youthful target audience and their parents. However, messengers are sometimes more effective outside their primary domains.

I don't usually lead the exercises in our DVDs, although I appear in

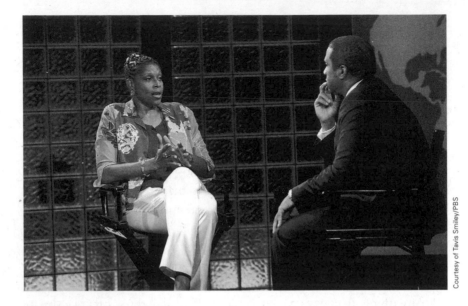

Courtesy of Tavis Smiley/PBS

Figure 14.   Dr. Yancey was interviewed by Tavis Smiley for a PBS obesity special in 2009.

all of them as an expert. The athletes and entertainers lead *Instant Recess*, and a lot of other regular folks lead the *Lift Off!*s. Being a doctor, former athlete, and 6-foot-2-inch woman, I garner respect for my professional accomplishments and represent a credible source of health information because of my training and intellect, but I'm neither a regular Jane nor a celebrity. If I develop a following among, say, baby boomers and women Gen Xers, I'll star in *Lift Off!*s aimed at those population segments. As evident from the volume of responses after our coverage on NPR and PBS, their early adopter audiences are taking note. It just underscores the point I find myself having to make over and over again: that it's not knowledge that drives behavior, but rather emotional connection.

The essence of marketing, social or commercial, is understanding the consumer—feeling, listening to, and connecting with your audience. How you think and what you create are very much products of your background and experiences, and there are no neutral observers. We all perceive the world through a cultural lens. If you don't understand the people you're trying to influence *in your bones*—if you don't get how they think or what they feel on a live-it, breathe-it, sleep-it level, you will not get traction no matter how broad your reach or high your visibility, penetration, or exposure. If you want your product or service to sell, you have to go to the people you're trying to reach. Don't expect them to come to you. If you're not a cultural insider, you'll have to do a lot more showing up to gain acceptance. But being a cultural insider doesn't give you an automatic pass. A third-generation college-educated Latino of Mexican heritage who learned Spanish in school is not necessarily going to be welcomed with open arms in a neighborhood of recent Mexican immigrants. And even if you grew up in that 'hood and moved away, you may still have a lot to learn about the current situation for people living there. You have to do some research. That's where focus groups, surveys, case studies and comparisons, and experiments come in. Do your homework on the competition so you can demonstrate the superiority of your offer. And when you get there, you damn straight better offer them something *they* want, not just something *you* think they need!

FIVE

The Case for the *Instant Recess* Model

Almost everybody wants to look and feel better. But in the long run the cost of doing so is high, the rewards are few and slow to materialize, and the obstacles are many. How often have we climbed that mountain against all odds, experiencing the elation of having achieved or nearly achieved a goal, and then plunged into the desperation, despair, or resignation accompanying our gradual or precipitous resumption of old habits when the odds caught up with us? Sure, it seems easy to take up a fitness regimen on your own—walking outdoors, say, is as cheap as a good pair of sneaks and can be very pleasant and uplifting if the weather's warm or crisp and sunny and the surroundings are appealing. But if you're middle aged and overweight and there are hills in either direction, a little rain might be just the excuse you need to stay in for a day or two. Especially since you were pretty gung ho on those first couple of days, and now your knees and thighs ache. You get back out there a few days later, but now the newness and euphoria after taking that first big step are wearing off, and your motivation comes in fits and starts. Life intrudes—it's always something. Your co-worker's car is in the shop and she needs a ride home. By the time you get home, it's starting to get chilly and dark, and your favorite show is on TV. You've got to drop the dogs off at the groomer's, your hairdresser has only one appointment available before your big presentation, your sinuses are bothering you, your sister's got comp tickets to a play you've been wanting to see, you have to work late, your kid's soccer game is this evening, your mom has a doctor's appointment . . . You look up and it's been a week since you hit the streets. You redouble your efforts and make it out the door for your walk every evening for the next week. Then your mom lands in the hospital for a week, and you look up and it's been a month since your last walk. You pick up a couple of pounds and you get out of breath more quickly next time. Your resolve wanes sooner or later under the onslaught of appealing sedentary options, and the spiraling time and energy demands in your busy life. Your exercise and healthy eating habits, despite your best intentions, eventually fall by the wayside.

The reason you so often start and stop exercise regimes is that you don't *build* the changes into your life. In other words, the reason you fail is that there's nothing shoring up your flagging, faltering, or just fickle motivation. How can you combat this? By tapping into the collective will, desire, and rapport of your friends, co-workers, bosses, colleagues, congregants, religious and political leaders, classmates, teachers, administrators, and partners and associates. Furthermore, injecting a little fun back into movement is essential if it's going to happen regularly. This is particularly true for women, since most were not socialized to develop skills for active recreation or to associate activity with femininity. *Instant Recess* is a starting point for those who've become overweight, out of shape, and essentially disconnected from really moving their bodies— who mostly equate exercise with drudgery, inadequacy, and boredom . . . in other words, the majority of Americans. "Treadmill" hasn't become a metaphor for nothing!

Research (mine and others') suggests that people of all backgrounds and body shapes respond favorably to introducing a little *recess* into their day, even those—especially those—not fond of moving and who're carrying more than a few extra pounds. Peer pressure, social comparisons and competition, and social support all come into play when you take a systems approach to fitness. If other people are doing it, you do it. "If Sally in the next cubicle can last those 10 minutes of a dance break— and Lord knows she's older and heavier than I am!—then I can, too." Everybody gets a good chuckle watching each other move and groove, puff and pant, slide and glide . . . those with rhythm and those without. The stress release and feelings of well-being carry over into the rest of the meeting or workday or service or class or event.

And peer pressure and competition operate at another level that spurs the adoption of recess breaks: between organizational leaders. If the interests of the organization are served and advanced along with those of the individual, that's a powerful incentive, whether it's a manufacturing plant, a clinic, a civic group, a school, a professional association, a church, a sports team, or a city. Better test scores, fewer disciplinary problems, more widgets, less spending on medical care and workers' comp, better equipped members, more enjoyable and better attended worship services, more loyal and committed fans, healthier and more engaged residents . . . these are much more powerful motivators for leaders than personal health and well-being are for most people. Why? Because in our work-obsessed society, social influences, cultural norms and values, incentives and rewards (like money and power), habits formed early in life, and survival instincts all line up to support investing in your career and doing a great job—at least at the upper managerial or executive level. Those not working outside the home are hardly exempt—there's a lot of pressure to be a good soccer mom or dad, and a lot of the scut work required to maintain home and hearth trickles, or more likely rushes, to those without a time clock to punch. That's hardly true for getting and staying fit. Images of lean and sexy people compete with those of sleek sedans and mesmerizing movies. Friends stroke you when you lose a few pounds and tempt you with sweets. The pull of the sofa and spectator sports on TV is so much stronger than the spinning class or the bike.

Everyone I know on the mature side of thirty-five, from dedicated athletes to equally committed couch and mouse potatoes, secretly or openly rues the encroaching inches of abdominal girth that most of us accumulate a bit each year. Everyone is getting bigger, even highly trained and fit professional athletes. The PAC 10 offensive linesmen today are about 50 pounds heavier on average than they were when I was a college athlete in the 1970s, and I thought they were really big back then! My social circles include a lot of trim former athletes, but rarely do I see anyone over forty without a bigger bulge in the middle than he or she desires, including what I see when *I* look down. Even folks like me, dedicated to finding the five or six hours each week to run or play in gyms and fields, on courts and roads, not infrequently fall short of our fitness goals, like that 10,000 daily step target. Modern society conspires against us at every turn, and we need to rely on each other to resist it. Fat or thin, athletic or uncoordinated, young or old, male or female, we *all* need a little (or a lot) more *recess* in our everyday lives. Every step counts! Every calorie expended is one that doesn't end up around our waists, so integrating more physical activity into our daily "conduct of business" benefits us all, as people, as organizations, and as a society.

THE CONCEPTUAL FRAMEWORK

The availability of environmental supports, like cheaper parking permits for remote lots, is critical, because many changes are not individually determined. Just envision federal regulatory mandates for daily exercise breaks on paid time. Think about the droves of people who successfully quit smoking and stayed quit, many with a number of previous failed attempts, once smoking was banned in their workplace, the cost of cigarettes skyrocketed, and others began to look at them with disdain or outright hostility. This led me to the concept of recess as a scalable and easily disseminated model for adding physical activity back into daily life in a changing society. There are many ways to systematically reinject activity into daily organizational routine, but I carefully designed my approach to incorporate research in the areas of marketing, social psychology, and innovation diffusion theory. I wound up with ten vital elements—the Ten Commandments of the recess model:

1. *Institutionalization.* Activity is part of the structure of the organization, occurring with regularity once or twice each day, with a prompt ingrained in all of us: the recess bell!

    Make the practice socially obligatory and target captive audiences. To get to people who aren't exercising—let's optimistically describe them as being at the "earlier stages in the fitness-related lifestyle-change continuum"—you have to make activity the default choice. They've demonstrated time and again that they're not going to do it on their own. It's apparently not worth going out of their way to participate. But make it obligatory and they'll say, "The boss says we all have to do it. And what the heck, it's better than feeding data into a spreadsheet."

2. *Compulsory opportunity.* Interruption of duties or lessons is mandatory, but active participation is not, mitigating feelings of coercion—You can lead a horse to water, but you can't make him *swim*.

    Develop strategies that rely less on individual volition and motivation. Supportive cultural values, substantial discretionary time or money, and widespread access to active leisure opportunities are the exception, not the rule, in our obesogenic society. These characteristics and constraints are not typical of ethnic minority and non-affluent communities, with their longer commutes, inconvenient public transit, less available high-quality child or elder care, distant or unaffordable fitness facilities, and less favorable attitudes toward exercise born of generations of being relegated to manual labor. So you have to start slowly and build steadily. Capitalize on the immediate positive effects of physical activity, like more energy, stress relief, and uplifted moods. Drawing the focus to these intrinsic reinforcements begins to relegate any participation incentives you've used to enhance the offer (see chapter 4) as secondary to their own positive feelings. With time, they'll experience the many longer-term benefits of being active. More substantial investments of time, money, and other resources will then be possible to further infuse and diffuse these changes in daily routine, both by individuals in their personal lives and by organizational decision makers.

3. *Ubiquity.* Recess activities can be done everywhere, by everybody, in any attire, crossing the lines of gender, race and ethnicity, socio-economic status, region, religion, and residence (urban, suburban, or rural).

    Everybody can participate but not necessarily in the same way—activity should be inescapable in some form or fashion. The captive audience of office workers is predominantly sedentary and overweight, unaccustomed to associating physical exertion with anything positive, so a gentle reintroduction is in order—*re*introduction, since most of us had fun when we were active as kids, and those memories and feelings can be reawakened. So encourage incremental change from a realistic baseline. Short bouts of group exercise can involve simple, low-impact, moderate-intensity movements requiring a manageable level of exertion with minimal risk of injury. However, they can be performed at higher levels of intensity by more fit individuals, thereby accommodating a range of agility, aerobic fitness, weight status, age, and functional ability levels. This means that everyone can participate to some degree, even if they do it on a chair. When I was leading an exercise break at the Milbank Boys and Girls Club in Harlem as a part of a launch event for the Professional Athletes Council, Rocket Ishmael, who used to play football for Notre Dame and several pro teams, said, "Wow, I can really feel that in my triceps!" And I can't tell you how many times I've been approached by people after leading an exercise break in a professional meeting and told that they actually enjoyed themselves—expressions like "I can actually do this, and wouldn't mind doing it again," or "I haven't had this much exercise in years!" or "I would never have done this if it wasn't part of the regular program, but it wasn't so bad!" and "I know I need to do something about my weight, but I didn't think I could without being no good for the rest of the day."

4. *Social interaction.* Peer pressure, social support, and role modeling by colleagues and leaders, invite active participation. Offering a variety of activities caters to a range of interests and tastes, often stratified by age or gender.

    We generally choose role models with whom we share characteristics like gender, class, ethnicity or—particularly when it comes to exercise—weight status and age, so recruit a diverse group of people as exercise leaders with whom others can identify and relate. Role models may enhance others' feelings of confidence and competency (inspirational—"If he can do it, I can do it"), or they may represent an ideal to strive for but not necessarily reach (aspirational—"I want to be like Mike"). I saw the power of social interaction and expectation in action on my own forty-eighth birthday. My partner, Darlene, not surprisingly also a very active person, is wonderfully creative at event planning, having been the development director of a small AIDS nonprofit. She surprised me with a "walking birthday party": about twenty friends came over for champagne and appetizers, and for dinner we proceeded to an Ethiopian restaurant that's about six blocks away. Believe me, we've got a lot of sedentary ex-jocks in our crowd who rarely walk a half mile at one time. Granted, it was hardly a brisk pace, but no one drove, and everyone made it there and back and had a great time doing it.

5. *Entertainment and amusement.* Physical exertion is placed in a positive and appealing light. The idea of it invokes fun—activities are eagerly anticipated and awaited each day, sometimes several times a day. ·

    Reframe the exercise as play, not work or drudgery—an entitlement to move rather than another dreaded obligation—in contrast to the dominant public perception of exercise. However, to be consistent with this notion of lightness and inclusiveness, deflect the focus away from weight loss and body image ideals. To work, the recess model must radiate acceptance and banish judgmental attitudes, which are just what people who perceive themselves to be unfit expect from those who are fit and trying to get them to be fit. Case in point—the ugly 2009 New Jersey governor's race made uglier by the incumbent's ridiculing his corpulent challenger in campaign ads with unflattering shots with the tagline, ". . . threw his weight around" (Halbfinger 2009). *Not* encountering those attitudes can be a pleasant surprise to less fit individuals, bolstering the chances for dissemination—they'll want to do it again, they'll request it, they'll talk about it, and they may even demonstrate a few moves for others. Not long ago, I sat beside a colleague, an African American woman carrying a few extra pounds, at a business awards breakfast. She confessed, only partly joking, that she had to watch what she ate because she was sitting next to a "fitness doctor." I assured her that I'm not the food police, and that it's because I enjoy eating that I try to get folks, me included, a little activity throughout the day. This seemed to reassure her, and she went on to tell me about the intimidation many of her young clients express at seeing nothing but painfully and unattainably thin people in the media. I told her that we deliberately show people, especially lean and fit ones like professional athletes, in loose clothing in our DVDs. This takes the spotlight off their amazing physiques and keeps the focus on the behavioral improvements that we can all make, regardless of our weight. My colleague subsequently asked me to help her incorporate recess-type physical activity into a number of her agency's youth programs for mostly overweight African American and Latino girls.

6. *Familiarity and distinction. Instant Recess* makes social marketing easier because people automatically "get it" in a single word that's unique in this regard—connoting activities, fun, and time out or relief from duty.

Make the concept memorable but simple and easily grasped by most people. There's a lot of competition for people's attention in our postmodern society, precisely because of the deluge of audiovisual, mostly electronic, stimuli as we move through the day. You can't pump gas, ride in a high-rise building elevator, or buy groceries these days without a screen showing a loop of commercials. It takes something a little off the beaten track to make people literally stand up and take notice. Sharon McDaniel-Lowe, a foundation CEO, was part of a small contingency from the board of directors of Casey Family Programs, a large Seattle-based foster care agency who visited me at my office to learn about my work. Another of its board members, Dr. America Bracho, a close collaborator who's one of my twin souls in a completely different package (a 5-foot-tall Venezuelan immigrant fireball) had persuaded them to consider a wellness initiative in their strategic planning and felt that the recess model might fill the bill. Of course, that meeting included an activity break. When I next ran into Sharon with a group of her colleagues, after I had led a recess break to kick off Casey's national conference, she turned to one of them and encouraged her to include "Dr. Toni's Stand Up, Get Off the Couch Butt Thing" at their next social work convening. One of the labels for the breaks is the *Lift Off!*—or *Lift* those buns *Off* the couches, and cheeks *Off* the chairs! Her amusing and slightly altered version speaks to the salience of the lighthearted packaging.

7. *Available facilities and space.* Usually gyms or playgrounds are dedicated for this purpose, but any convenient and accessible space will do, indoors or out.

   Instant Recess breaks can be done anywhere, anytime, by anybody, in any attire. This makes them manageable in settings with prohibitive resource constraints—of space, fitness equipment, or outdoor surroundings conducive to activity (weather, safety, and appeal). Portable technology can convert any meeting room, lobby, or foyer into a festive spot for a little activity. Computer software prompts or broadcast voice mail blasts can summon co-workers to fitness breaks or walking meetings, and word processing software automated reminders are extremely powerful and handy tools. Social networking Web sites like Facebook can also be used to spread the word. If it can be used to help elect an African American president, it can be used to get people to exercise.

8. *Cultural congruence and adaptability.* Similar and different activities take place in Kansas, Kentucky, Kensington, and Kauai.

Target and build on community strengths and assets. Not only are CDs and DVDs turnkey instructional tools, but they can also incorporate images, sounds, and personalities that have cultural meaning and resonance, like hip-hop music and professional athletes to target urban schools and youth programs, gospel music and aerobics to engage black churches, and mega-church televangelists and progressive country music to reach Southern whites in the Bible Belt. The cultural salience of dance and music and the collectivism (where family and social obligation trumps individualism) among African Americans, American Indians, Asian Americans, Pacific Islanders, and Latinos—for whom dancing at parties is normal even in middle and older age—represents an opportunity.

9. *Carryover or spillover to other venues.* Recess often introduces kids to activities they like or are suited to.

I'd never been good at any sport—could barely walk and chew bubble gum at the same time given how fast I was growing—until I happened upon a tetherball game one recess period in fifth grade. I realized that, long-limbed at 5 feet 7 inches, once I got the ball, no one else could touch it! Of course, a tetherball set quickly topped my Christmas list and provided afternoon and weekend fun for me and my posse for several years. *Instant Recess* breaks are an opportunity for people to rediscover that physical exertion can be enjoyable, to be reminded of the fun they're missing out on. I often see a youthful light gleaming from the eyes of a middle-aged former athlete run to seed when doing a batting (baseball) or shooting (basketball) or catching and cutting (football) move from one of the *Instant Recess* breaks. They're also a sort of wake-up call to remind people they've gotten a bit out of shape. Several times I've been stopped by colleagues who'd previously attended a lecture or meeting in which I'd led recess breaks; they share that they'd not realized how much their fitness had slipped until they got out of breath after only 5 minutes. They began walking, joined a gym or reupped a lapsed membership, or found a tennis or racquetball partner. On an organizational level, you can capitalize on the ripple effect that one decision by a leader has on many others. People at all levels within an organization or in the broader society choose leaders for a reason—they follow because there's something about that person that they admire or want to emulate, so the head of a corporation influences her executive team, who influence the middle managers, who influence the supervisors, who influence the line staff. And the bosses brag about their (personal and organizational) results at professional meetings, civic gatherings, and country clubs, influencing other decision makers, and at some point, ultimately legislative and regulatory policy makers.

10. *Reinforcement of the mission.* Market *Instant Recess* in a way that supports the mission of the organization.

Ultimately, any innovation must assist in meeting core business goals, not just health goals. For example, managing staff stress loads in hard economic times may be emphasized for human services agencies; savings to the bottom line from lower patient complication rates or medication needs, for medical managed care groups; or enhanced productivity and less attrition (lowering training costs), in for-profit corporations. A prime example of conveying consistency with mission is the recent academic push to demonstrate definitively that time spent in physical activity delivers a spectrum of benefits for students, teachers, and administrators. Interest in getting *Instant Recess* and similar interventions back into the schools has been driven by the childhood obesity epidemic, but in fact, studies show that physical activity measurably improves academic performance, the core mission of schools. It's interesting to me that the decline in boys' academic persistence and performance (girls now comprise more than 60 percent of college students, and the percentage is even higher among African Americans and Latinos) has paralleled the creeping sedentariness of the school day.

HOW DOES IT WORK?

Implementing any new practice or policy comes down to the components and the channels through which they operate, marketing and communications, participation incentives, evaluation mechanisms, and financial or budget implications. For *Instant Recess*, the upfront investment, start-up costs, and long-term commitments are negligible.

Several things have to happen to get *Instant Recess* up and going in a workplace, school, or other organizational setting where people spend a lot of time. First, the leaders must communicate clearly that the changes represent a benefit rather than an obligation and reflect management concern about their well-being. This takes buzz or viral marketing among the rank and file that this effort is different from the others management may have put into play. It also requires talking with a few well-respected workers from different levels of the company hierarchy before *Instant Recess* breaks are implemented, to help figure out the best way to go about this. Second, it will take multiple "recess champions" of two types: fitness enthusiasts comfortable in leading group exercises, and opinion leaders to whom others look for assurance and guidance as "keepers" of the work culture, usually older women fairly senior but low in the hierarchy of the organization. Few individuals fit both criteria, but both types are necessary. Ideally, champions are identified through self-referral or co-worker recommendation, not management assignment. You need several in each category for sustainability to offset the inevitable attrition or changes in job assignments over time. Champions publicize and encourage participation by employees or members, help to set new norms and expectations, lead daily activity breaks, communicate updates regularly using existing channels, stay alert for new resources and fresh ideas, advocate for the program, and innovate to better fit the organizational culture and to keep the program from getting stale or humdrum.

For example, the Los Angeles Urban League was one of the organizations in our UCLA worksite pilot study. At one of its child care facilities, after several weeks of incorporating a "standard" daily aerobic dance exercise break, it branched out to tailor the program for its own work environment. The youthful Gen Y staffers created a variety of exercise breaks: they ran obstacle courses, played "basketball" games with a large exercise ball, and did aerobics videos and audiotapes. They displayed a remarkable facility with current information technology by downloading "old school" soul and disco concert footage from YouTube and choreographing group dances to "Thriller," "Cupid Shuffle," and "Payaso de Rodeo." Ideally, there's a wellness coordinator to whom these activities fall naturally. We've generally found them to be quite receptive, extremely helpful in functioning as a liaison between their agencies and our research staff, and enthusiastically supportive. But since wellness coordinators are few and far between in most small and medium-sized nonprofits and businesses, these duties must become institutionalized as a part of somebody's job description. Most volunteers eventually tire of these responsibilities once the newness wears off and their regular duties more often get in the way.

Last, buy-in and visible support from the top must be ongoing. Managers must regularly participate in group activities when their schedules permit, and they must ensure that staff who assume responsibility for incorporating the changes are allowed time for training and ongoing technical assistance. My buddy Jim Sallis brought back a great idea from a leading physical activity researchers' shop in New Zealand to break up the endless hours of sitting in meetings. A professor at San Diego State University, Jim heads the Robert Wood Johnson Foundation's Active Living Research Program. He probably has more claim to fame than anyone else as a modern luminary of population physical activity promotion. At the foundation's 2009 national meeting, he introduced the standing ovation as the standard show of appreciation after a talk. It certainly makes the speaker feel good and, most importantly, gets those cheeks off the chairs.

The key ingredient is "regularizing" the changes—making them part of the way business is done. Here's a list of model core and elective practices and policies.

CORE ("PUSH" STRATEGIES)

- Incorporate 10-minute exercise breaks during lengthy meetings and at a scheduled time of the day. (*Lift Off!*s or *Instant Recess* breaks).
- Restrict nearby parking to the disabled and provide incentives for distant parking.
- Make standing ovations, instead of sitting and clapping, the standard show of appreciation for speakers.
- Support other individual and group exercises during the routine "conduct of business"—hold walking meetings, for example, and schedule sit-down meetings in locations at a short distance from attendees' workspaces.
- Post stair prompts and ask managers and execs to take the lead in using the stairs instead of the elevator.
- Include healthy food choices at meetings in which refreshments are served (guidelines can be found at http://www.5colorsaday.com/, http://www.sph.umn.edu/news/nutritionalguidelines, and http://www.uhs.berkeley.edu/facstaff/healthmatters/healthymeetings.shtml).
- Include at least 50 percent healthy and competitively priced food choices in workplace vending machines, cafeterias, and on-site food vendor offerings.
- Adopt formal written policies institutionalizing these practices and informal policies.
- Include wellness policy implementation duties in the job descriptions of senior managers *and* line or administrative staff. Such duties would include organizing and coordinating activity breaks and walking meetings, securing physical activity and nutrition-promotion materials, handling the purchase and delivery of water and fruit/nut snacks, and ensuring adherence to food-procurement policy.
- Change the organizational culture to promote and reward lifestyle activity, including standing up at intervals, doing "airline" exercises in one's chair, stretching during meetings.

- Replace candy and cookie jars on organizational leaders' (and preferably all employees') desks with bowls of fruit or small packages (no more than 2 ounces) of nuts (preferably unsalted) or dried fruit/nut mix.
- Establish healthy food procurement and fund-raising policies for catering and conference and meeting facility menus.

ELECTIVE ("MENU OF OPTIONS")

- Encourage more casual attire compatible with lifestyle integration of physical activity; for example, relegate neckties and high-heeled shoes to formal or special occasions, not everyday wear (as the daily expectation or norm).
- Provide a bowl of fresh fruit in the reception or central congregating area.
- Link networked computers to a printer at a distance from employees' workspace to necessitate a short walk (three to five minutes).
- Install water fountains or dispensers.
- Replace desk and conference chairs with stability balls (including stands to protect novice users).
- Improve stairwell appeal and accessibility, and discourage elevator use by slowing them and skipping floors.
- Include language in subcontracts mandating or providing incentives for suppliers' adoption of healthy/fit practices and policies.
- Provide substantive incentives for mass transit use.
- Establish automobile-free zones around schools, workplaces, and shopping areas. Move employee or student "drop-off" locations sufficiently far from workplace or school entrances to require at least a five- to ten-minute walk to work or class.
- Encourage the acquisition of dogs to prompt walking during nonwork hours, for example, by hosting adoption fairs by rescue organizations on site.

Getting something going and *keeping* it going are two different things. Nico Pronk, my co-author on a work-site wellness book chapter whose focus is on the private sector, talks about the four Ss, a simple set of rules that combine science and practice to capture the realities of program design and implementation: *size, scope, scalability,* and *sustainability*

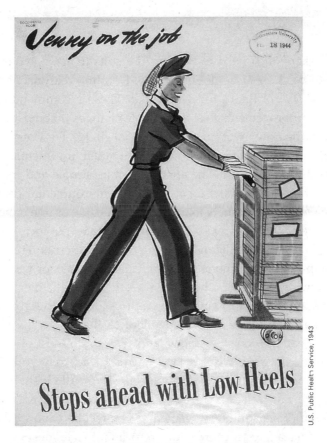

Figure 15.   From a WWII public ad campaign, "Jenny on the Job" demonstrates beauty and fashion taking a back seat to health and safety.

(Yancey, Pronk, and Cole 2007). I'll address these when describing the unfolding of the recess model in the next chapter. However, since participation is one of the most important early indicators of success, it may be useful to highlight a few ways of securing rank-and-file buy-in, such as including union leaders in planning, making special outreach efforts to those low on the totem pole (usually where ethnic minority workers are concentrated), and visibly reflecting inclusiveness of medically at-risk groups like obese, disabled, or older people.

HOW CAN *YOU* MAKE IT WORK?

Adult workers don't need to wait for the suits to act. Anyone can take action—at work or at home. In table 1, I outline reasonably easy concrete steps that ordinary folks can take. These recommendations link individual improvements to small, doable changes that most people can manage in their own workplaces and social circles. For every successful personal lifestyle change, there should be an environmental change to *anchor* that new behavior. The anchors can be simple and inexpensive. Recess breaks can take the form of social environmental changes like getting your choir members to insert a brief gospel or line dance session into their weekly rehearsals. They can also take the form of physical changes, like setting daily midmorning and midafternoon reminders on your computer or cell phone to prompt recess breaks or walking meetings. But there are lots of other anchors—the more, the merrier!

It's vital for people just embarking on this journey to start with many small steps, none of which are dependent on the others. For example, if you set a goal of 8,000 steps a day, and plan to do most of those at the gym before you go to work in the morning, each day you either win the lottery or go bankrupt. If you get to the gym, all's well. If you don't, though, you fall far short of the minimum level of activity necessary for the kind of waistline you want, and you feel bad about your lack of progress. Instead, restructure your program into a modest *daily paycheck* by spreading out the opportunities to squeeze in those 8,000 steps. You can get 1,500 steps in a 10 a.m. walking meeting, 2,000 to and from work by buying the cheaper parking permit in the remote lot, 2,000 during the course of the workday during brief group fitness breaks, and another 1,000 in the union meeting over which you're presiding tonight, having placed a movement break on the agenda. With the 1,500 to 2,000 steps you get from daily household chores, you've more than met the goal! Even if the alarm clock breaks, traffic is bad, or you get called to that unexpected morning meeting, you're still almost there, and you're more likely to summon up the energy even at the end of the long day to walk the dog for ten minutes to make up those steps—and you'll have more energy to summon because you took all those steps earlier in the day. If

Table 1 Ten ways to anchor your individual lifestyle changes in organizational supports

Your move	Anchor
Take an *Instant Recess* break every four hours in the form of a structured 10-minute movement break or a quick stroll around the office or grounds, or a lively salsa dance session.	Incorporate or instigate the integration of *Instant Recess* breaks in meetings lasting an hour or longer, and schedule at least one walking meeting each week. Set an electronic organizer, a cell phone, or a computer reminder to prompt a *Lift Off!* at your work station or desk. Better yet, get the OK for a midmorning and midafternoon booster break with music and voiceover broadcast throughout the office over the intercom system, and post reminders for your co-workers of the time for the break in the lunchroom or break room. Or send out a broadcast e-mail message announcement!
Drink eight to ten or more 8-ounce glasses of water per day, and curtail your caffeine. The only other beverage I drink, besides an occasional beer or glass of champagne, is a pint of unstrained fresh-pressed carrot juice or other veggie juice combo every day or two—see below.	Water is healthy, fills you up, has no calories, and may even help you burn a few. Purchase a water dispenser for your own office for convenience and a constant visual reminder and behavioral prompt. Better yet, get your co-workers to chip in on the dispenser. Best of all, get your employer to subsidize the dispenser. Along with exercise, water and plant fiber decrease the time that waste stays in your system and may take a few calories along with it. Ask your vendor truck operator, grocer, or cafeteria manager to stock fresh veggie juice, if they don't already. Request that the sodas be relegated to the periphery of the vending machines, with the low-fat milk, fruits, 100% veggie juices, and water in the central eye-level slots. Solicit your employer to subsidize the carrot juice so that it's less expensive or no more costly than the less nutritious selections.

(continued)

you do get to the gym, that's a bonus for your waistline, but if not, you've still burned a few calories and given your mood and immune system a boost without *sweating it*.

And don't forget that you have to fuel up to lift off! Water intake through drinking water and eating foods high in water content like

Table 1 (continued)

Your move	*Anchor*
Eat at least five colors of fruits and veggies each day. The federal recommendation is five to nine servings—a serving is the amount you can hold in your hand—per day, but five colors is a lot easier to remember.	Place a bowl of fresh fruit or jar of dried fruit on your desk at work or in a common reception area. Take turns with your colleagues procuring this produce from farmers' or other locally grown produce markets. Better yet, get your employer to subsidize the communal fruit bowl, arrange delivery of boxes of fresh produce, or co-locate a farmers' market at your job site, like certain Kaiser Permanente locations. Ask restaurant waitstaff to remove bread or tortilla chips as munchies, substituting celery and carrot sticks or edamame (baby soybeans in a green pod) or jicama chopped into bite-sized morsels with salsa or pico de gallo dip.
Fidget frequently.	Engage the most vocal co-workers or opinion leaders where you work to shift the work culture to frown upon long periods of sitting "chained to your desks," to establish pedometer wearing as a cultural norm, to support standing and stretching during meetings, and to discourage the wearing of neckties and high-heeled shoes, which discourage lifestyle integration of physical activity during the workday.
Reduce the amount of fat, sugar, refined grains, and salt you consume in one meal or snack, and increase your vegetable intake. Beware of supersizing!	Replace your dinner plate with a salad plate for meals at home—they're the same size as 1950s dinner plates. Purchase convenience or snack foods in one- or two-serving packages. Place fruits and vegetables most conspicuously in the refrigerator and the pantry; chop them into bite-sized pieces and store in clear plastic containers so they are as convenient as highly processed snacks. Place high-calorie desserts or snacks out of easy reach and eyesight. Ask for a takeout container at the beginning of the meal when dining out, and package a third to a half of your entree and dessert before eating. Always order a non-cream-based vegetable soup or garden salad with the dressing on the side when dining out to blunt the appetite and lessen your devouring bread or other calorie-dense appetizers.

Table 1

Your move	Anchor
Walk up at least one and down at least two flights of stairs whenever your indoor or outdoor activities permit.	Post stair prompts at your workplace and in other buildings you frequent near elevators. Lead co-workers to the stairs instead of the elevators when travelling in groups at work. Engage your workplace wellness committee or coordinator in increasing stair appeal and access and restricting elevator access and convenience (for example, through skip-stop or hydraulic elevators).
Bring vegetable- or fruit-based dishes to work and social potlucks.	Advocate for healthy food procurement policies at your worksite and in other organizations to which you belong. Instigate the inclusion of healthy and tasty food choices in vending machines; as refreshments at work and at social meetings and events; and among vendor selections at work, in groceries you patronize, and in buildings you frequent.
Wear a pedometer like you wear a watch, consulting it frequently.	Invest in an accurate and reliable, research-quality pedometer to allow intensity recording and seven-day storage of step counts. (Cheaper models are less sensitive to movement and tend to undercount steps.)
Park farther away from your destinations as you work, shop, play, worship, and socialize. Make short utilitarian trips (for groceries) on foot or bike. Use mass transit at least once a week if possible.	Purchase a parking space in a distant lot and request a discount from your employer for doing so. Buy a monthly bus or train pass to prompt a certain minimum monthly usage to avoid wasting money. If available, identify and take advantage of, or establish employer-supported incentives for, active commuting (mass transit, walking, biking).
Schedule seven to eight hours of sleep per night, and protect that time.	Purchase window treatments to ensure adequate darkness of the bedroom, located, if possible, in a quiet part of the house, removed from traffic noises, or those of family members with different sleeping schedules. Install double-pane windows and carpeting in nearby or overhead rooms if necessary to mute unavoidable noise disturbances. Invest in a high-quality mattress. Restrict the amount of light emitted by clocks and other electronic devices. (You can house them inside cabinets or unplug them when not in use. Buy a power strip to make it easy—just a flip of a switch that also saves you money and takes a bite out of your carbon footprint.) Ideally, remove the TV from the bedroom (I haven't quite gotten there yet).

fruits and veggies gives your skin a nice glow, alleviates strain on your kidneys, and is necessary to burn fat—along with lots of other health benefits. In addition to maintaining a high level of energy output, I attribute much of my ability to maintain a healthy body weight over time to not *drinking* any calories other than veggie juice and the occasional herb tea, beer, or glass of champagne. Sodas, lattes, cappuccinos, and other caloric drinks have little nutritional value and are deadly for the waistline! Sodas also deplete your bones of calcium and may speed bone thinning. Most importantly, they're dehydrating, not hydrating—sort of defeats the purpose of drinking in the first place.

I have a few other things going for me, eating-wise. I haven't eaten beef or pork in twenty-five years, and I eat whole grains whenever possible, often passing on white breads and pastas. I try to eat a rainbow of colors every day. I love tomatoes in all forms and put salsa or chunky tomato sauce, along with spinach, in just about everything I cook. I'm a bean lover from way back—black-eyed peas, navy beans, black beans, green and yellow split peas, you name 'em. And I was taught the joys of cooking with soy by the best—I make a mean scrambled tofu and soy bacon dish that most people confuse for the real thing. I think Michael Pollan (2006) has it about right: "Eat food. Not too much. Mostly plants." Of course, I don't always get it right. My Achilles' heel is dairy. I've a lifelong deep and abiding love—a real jones for ice cream and frozen yogurt, cheese of most varieties, sour cream in my chili and on my quesadillas and chilaquiles, and whipped cream in my soy hot chocolate. I've adored macaroni and cheese since childhood! I make it a little differently from scratch—with whole wheat pasta and soy milk, but I regularly succumb to temptation from the real McCoy, especially since that's our granddaughter's favorite dish. Fortunately, adult-onset lactose intolerance slowed me down in my late thirties. But that's where activity comes in.

So my mantra's something like, "Be active. Not too little. Mostly low impact." The last is a pretty recent phenomenon, wrought by my terrible genetic predisposition for early onset and rapidly progressive osteo-arthritis I mentioned earlier, now manifesting in stiffness after sitting even five minutes, four knee surgeries, a lot of creakiness, and even more when I forget to take my glucosamine and chondroitin. My attitude is, when you pass fifty, you're going to spend more time with your cardiologist or your orthopedist. I like my orthopod and much prefer bad joints to a bad heart!

And here's another unrelated tidbit. Install a full-length mirror on your closet or bathroom door. My hairdresser, Kenny, is a singer-actor a little younger than me with a bad family history of diabetes, which he's escaped so far by losing 80 pounds from a high of 300. We somehow started lamenting the amount of time and money many women are willing to spend on their appearance—hair, makeup, manicures, pedicures, and shoes—but are unwilling to spend on getting their bodies in shape. He chalked it up to "shrinking mirror syndrome," looking only at their faces or hands or feet, but not at their whole bodies. That resonated with me, not only because of the sobering image staring back at me in the mirror, hardly the svelte-model visage from an earlier life, but also because of a story that Octavia (my friend and project manager) told me when we first met. In her early fifties, she said, she got her wake-up call—which ultimately led to her running marathons—in a hotel bathroom with those huge mirrors that catch your whole body from every angle. She claims she startled herself as she stepped into the shower because she thought her reflection was an intruder!

So, add fun to the mix, make fitness a system, and don't put all your eggs in one basket. In other words, give yourself a lot of opportunities for things to go right without a huge investment of time and energy. Human inertia is a daily reality, both (1) literally—it's much harder to get out of the house to go to the gym once you've gotten home and settled in than it is to stop off on the way home from work, and (2) conceptually—dramatic lifestyle changes usually end quickly (unless precipitated by a heart attack or cancer diagnosis). But incremental or insidious changes sneak up on you. They then become habits and are more easily sustained over the long haul.

IS IT WORKABLE?

Yes, I've personally facilitated thousands of recess breaks during the past decade in a variety of situations, including grant review committees and lecture presentations for the American Cancer Society and National

Institutes of Health, boards of directors meetings, government hearings, monthly meetings of local health coalitions and medical and public health societies, and local, state, and national public health, medical, and mental health conferences. And once, even, stuck in a snowstorm on the way to a social marketing conference in Lake Tahoe.

Despite some initial hesitancy, the participation rates have usually been over 90 percent, with only a few folks skating out the back door. I've gotten many very favorable unsolicited comments. One heavyset individual in Houston, Texas, told us it was "the most exercise I've had in ten years!" Another said, "I feel that I am finally doing something for myself . . . taking charge of my health." Typical was Donald Felder's response. A stocky social worker at the Casey Family Programs annual meeting in Seattle in January 2009, he rushed up to me, energized, and said simply, "I can do this!" He proceeded to tell me that he was going to lead a recess break at a meeting with school administrators the following week and convince principals that it needed to be in all the schools . . . and should be happening everywhere.

I didn't always have ringing endorsements from the folks running things. As a self-designated "boisterous leader," however, I've come to realize that I drive a lot more change when I ask for forgiveness rather than permission. And now, of course, people know what to expect when they see me coming—and I usually get a very enthusiastic reception!

Best of all, the strategy seems to be gaining traction well outside my sphere of influence. LuAnn Heinen, whom I interviewed for this book in her role as an executive in the National Business Group on Health, mentioned that a recent federal quality assurance meeting included an exercise video clip embedded in the slide show that got everyone up and moving. Daily stretching exercises at the beginning of the day are not uncommon in progressive companies where the work involves physical labor. My Head Diva in Charge, my assistant Danielle, caught an episode of a Discovery Channel show around Labor Day in 2004 featuring a construction company that mandated stretching routines before starting work on a Northern California Bay Bridge project. I'll get back to this in more detail in the next chapter.

To more systematically evaluate the feasibility of *Instant Recess*, our

UCLA research team, with help from colleagues at other institutions, surveyed an ethnically diverse group of 137 professionals at public health conferences or training seminars at which exercise breaks were conducted in Los Angeles and Monterey, California; Dallas and Houston, Texas; and Atlanta, Georgia. They thought the program was a great idea. On average, they ranked the idea of having exercise breaks in longer meetings a fantastic idea (4.6 points out of 5) and the feasibility of workplace exercise breaks "easily doable" (4.4 points out of 5). Participants said they were relatively confident that they could lead an exercise break (after being trained) and host a walking meeting (each 7.5 of 10). Overall, 96 percent of the respondents endorsed the exercise break as a good or great concept. Yes, these were public health professionals, so they may be preconditioned, but I assure you that, on the whole, they're in no better shape than the rest of the population. It's apparent at any conference of nutritionists, nurses, physicians, or other health professionals that *knowing* better is not synonymous with *doing* better!

Then, we partnered with researchers at other universities and looked at diverse groups of lay people, including nurses, teachers, and church members in different regions of the country, including the South, Midwest, and Northeast. They strongly agreed that exercise breaks are a good use of workday time and of their own time (4.55 and 4.36 of 5, respectively) and that, on average, they would like to participate in these breaks three times per week.

HOW TO GET IT TO WORK IN *YOUR* ORGANIZATION

Let's say you've started the process of getting you and your co-workers in your immediate vicinity moving, with the blessing of your boss. Your friends and enemies in other areas of the company are getting jealous of the fun y'all seem to be having, and you'd like to start testing the waters farther afield. Your boss is getting some positive strokes from her supervisors about what's happening, and you're happy with the chance to take it on the road and escape your cubicle a bit more often. How do you move forward? To give you a little guidance, I've assembled several profiles of different types of organizations that took that next step as part of our federally funded UCLA pilot study to formally evaluate *Instant Recess* and other "push" strategies.

Contrast the experiences of the Whittier Health Center, a county public health clinic in Whittier, California, and the county's Maternal, Child, and Adolescent Health Program, to those of Crystal Stairs, a community-based child care services and advocacy agency in Los Angeles. I've also included the profiles of two other types of organizations, a sorority and a church, to give you a feel for how the model works when the majority of participants are members, rather than employees. All of these organizations have strong and supportive leadership and a natural alignment of their own mission with our recess model wellness practices and policies.

Profile 1. Whittier Health Center

LOGISTICS

Whittier Health Center has eighty-six employees, approximately 40 percent of whom stay in the office while 60 percent regularly engage in field work. The staff is a mix of clinical providers, business, clerical, public health, and administrative managers. The facility operates on two floors, with staff equally distributed between them.

IMPLEMENTATION

Three program champions participated in the large, centrally hosted training session for representatives of multiple sites. They also requested on-site training for program champions for five additional staff members, including a decision maker for the facility. The project was interwoven into preexisting wellness endeavors: the WHC wellness committee spun off a subcommittee tasked with carrying out the details of planning and implementation. A key member of the subcommittee served as a liaison between WHC and UCLA. An implementation plan was crafted by the subcommittee and approved by the facility leader in short order. Within two weeks of the on-site staff training, the launch event occurred during a general staff meeting, such that participation in the first activity break was over 90 percent, including managers and senior staff. Ten-minute activity breaks were conducted twice daily nearly every day of the week. Participation rates fluctuated between ten and fifteen employees (about a quarter of the staff present), with some employees opting to participate in both breaks. Reminder announcements were broadcast over the intercom system at ten and five minutes before each activity break.

MAINTENANCE

Troubleshooting and problem solving were ongoing, as hosting breaks in upstairs and downstairs locations simultaneously was complicated by logistics. A decision was expeditiously made to focus efforts downstairs, and the upstairs staff was encouraged to participate. For variety when existing CDs and DVDs became mundane, champions devised a moderate-impact, continuous aerobic activity break modeled after three cultural group "party" line dances popular among clinic employees, with overwhelmingly positive response. Five- or ten-minute activity breaks were featured as a line item on the agenda of all general staff meetings in which WHC participated, including those of all surrounding feeder clinics, with employees from these satellite sites also expected to participate in the exercises.

THEMES AND CONSIDERATIONS

The staff used existing wellness infrastructure without the need to reinvent the wheel. The active support and participation of key decision makers was critical to implementation and maintenance. Responsibilities of the program champions were distributed among several employees. Creativity and adaptability were used in anticipating problems and refreshing intervention elements.

Profile 2. LA County Maternal, Child, and Adolescent Health Program

LOGISTICS

The Maternal, Child, and Adolescent Health Program has about seventy-five full- and part-time staff, 90 percent of whom are women, and more than 80 percent of whom spend the vast majority of their working hours at the headquarters facility. The multidisciplinary team includes physicians, public health nurses, policy analysts, administrators, nutritionists, health educators, social workers, research analysts, epidemiologists, data systems analysts, and support staff, organized into several work groups and units. The program is headquartered in a large multisuite floor of a high-rise consisting of multiple aisles of cubicles and several managerial office spaces.

IMPLEMENTATION

A 10-minute daily physical activity break is conducted every day at 4 p.m. Breaks are conducted in a central location, usually a large conference room to facilitate the use of CDs and DVDs, with an open hallway area as a backup when necessary. Participation rates average between ten and fifteen employees, or 15 to 20 percent of the total staff at any given break. Two program champions are formally charged with facilitating the breaks. Most units convene individually on a weekly basis for meetings and other activities, at which exercise breaks are routinely included. Quarterly all-staff "community-wide" meetings also feature breaks on the regular agenda, with 90 percent participation of the 100 to 120 attendees. The program has utilized the full library of *Instant Recess/Lift Off!* CDs and DVDs. CDs were preferred due to the minimal investment of time necessary to facilitate the activity. However, over time, these recordings have been replaced, for the most part, by a more goal-oriented commercial "walk for life" DVD found online and purchased by the workers. That break involves walking in place for 10 to 15 minutes to accumulate a mile a day or five miles a week, and for those having achieved a higher level of fitness, "boosted walking" (race walking or slow jogging) for bonus mileage accrual over the final 2 minutes of the break.

MAINTENANCE

A primary factor in the successful institutionalization of the breaks, from the program director's perspective, is the enthusiasm of the participants—their collective sense of taking action proactively to protect and enhance their health—and the recognition and appreciation they accord the program champions for their facilitation efforts. Active engagement by participants from the outset in choosing a regular time and selecting and trying out different types of exercise breaks staves off boredom and reinforces a sense of accomplishment and ownership. Program champions are fairly highly placed within the program hierarchy, so staff members respond readily to their authority. Ongoing leadership support is concretely reflected in the director's participation whenever she's present in the workplace (about every other week) and in the routine scheduling of breaks during all-staff meetings. When faced with challenges, managers have been very responsive and helpful in troubleshooting and finding solutions.

THEMES AND CONSIDERATIONS

Cultural as well as logistical issues figured into the choice of the time of day for the break: (1) most employees go home right after the break so that they don't worry about perspiration-related disturbances of clothing, hair, makeup, or body odor; and (2) the conference room is frequently booked during the middle of the workday, and employees like to have the option of playing DVDs, which they are not able to do earlier. Leadership has been critical at multiple levels, including the empowerment of staff participants to take responsibility and ownership of the implementation process.

Profile 3. Crystal Stairs

LOGISTICS

This agency has 350 employees distributed across four locations within a ten-mile radius. The employee mix includes business, clerical, social work, child care, and administrative managerial staff—full time, part time, seasonal, and volunteers. Administrative headquarters are housed in a multistory building, with staff located on several floors. The majority spend the workday in that facility.

IMPLEMENTATION

Several program champions from headquarters and satellite sites participated in the centrally hosted training session, but no on-site trainings were requested or provided. A huge launch event was attended by most headquarters staff and hosted in a central courtyard area as a health fair, with nutrient-rich foods, disease screening, and trainers from a nearby private fitness club offering free short-term memberships. Twice daily (except Friday), 10-minute activity breaks are offered in a central courtyard area, which requires a few minutes' walk and coming downstairs for most employees. Employees initiated a "Biggest Loser" contest within the first few months after launch, independently of UCLA (or Crystal Stairs management), conflicting with the recess model's de-emphasis on weight loss.

MAINTENANCE

Major funding cuts required sweeping layoffs six months after the intervention initiation, essentially eliminating the opportunity to collect follow-up data.

THEMES AND CONSIDERATIONS

Instant Recess breaks were readily institutionalized in child care sites, with kids serving as environmental prompts—as is true for school recess, they consistently remind staff at the appointed time and thoroughly enjoy the interludes. The decentralized agency setup led to a dilution of resources, both those provided by UCLA and those available from the agency. This was mostly reflected in program champion fatigue and overload (insufficient numbers at headquarters and at two sites, though adequate at the other). Secular commercial media-driven weight-loss competition fads created challenges in communications between sites within the agency, and between the agency and UCLA, which made it difficult to put the horse back in barn and advocate for "waist loss" versus weight-loss competitions. This was compounded by the lack of an existing wellness infrastructure, in that there was no mechanism for vetting health-related activities. In addition, the lower-level positioning of program champions within the agency hierarchy presented difficulties in the seating of authority and decision making. Last, fluctuating staffing requirements and modest workforce levels due to absences during flu season and holiday periods were complicated by frequent "all hands on deck" demands—for example, when large grant proposals or year-end reports were due.

It's apparent that Whittier and the Maternal, Child, and Adolescent Health Program, as local government facilities, are buffered to some extent from economic fluctuations, while Crystal Stairs, though government regulated and largely government funded (at least the service-delivery component), is still a freestanding private nonprofit agency. Its scope of operation and its resource availability are more closely tied to economic and political flux.

The critical difference in sustainability, as I noted, has likely been the greater fiscal stability of a government agency compared with that of a private nonprofit in an economic downturn, affecting staffing levels and morale. Instability presented communications difficulties—between champions and their co-workers, between champions at different locations in supporting each other, and between champions and UCLA. Another distinction was the alteration in the captive-audience aspect of the recess model. Decentralization in general created this deviation, both within headquarters and at satellite sites. For example, hosting breaks in the courtyard at headquarters made it easier to avoid them than participate in them—out of sight, out of mind. This limited opportunities to influence the organizational culture and institutionalize practice and policy changes.

Profile 4. My Sister's Keeper:
Delta Sigma Theta Sorority, Los Angeles

Another type of organization ripe for recess model policy change is the professional association or network. Graduate chapters of sororities in most black communities are a combination social and civic group. Their members are well educated and relatively affluent, but generally well connected to, and involved with, the larger black community. In addition, they tend to be concentrated in decision-making human services positions as administrators, clinicians, or leaders of nonprofits. There's obviously less infrastructure to build on—a few meetings a month instead of daily contact, but these associations present a great opportunity for exposing like-minded people to a wellness approach that might be useful in other contexts and venues.

The Los Angeles alumnae chapter of the national Delta Sigma Theta sorority has eighty members ranging in age from twenty-three to seventy-four years. There is an executive committee and seventeen standing committees, each with funding to support various activities. There is at least one general membership meeting and one executive committee meeting each month. While one of the committees is charged with health outreach activities, the organization has embraced a number of internal fitness-promoting practices and policies. The centerpiece changes are conducting physical activity breaks every two to three hours during meetings and events and enforcing healthy food procurement guidelines (supporting caterers offering whole grains, low-fat proteins, fruits, and veggies). Only nutrient-rich food purchases for standing committee meetings and activities are reimbursed—chips and sodas are on a member's own dime.

Cultural adaptations have been developed to address a major barrier to exercise for black women—hair maintenance. For example, the air conditioning is dialed down to lower the temperature in the room ten minutes before activity breaks to minimize perspiration and hair disturbance. Other wellness activities include instituting walking clubs at local high schools and recruiting organizational partners to provide support and fitness-promoting incentives such as yoga mats, pedometers, cooking classes, and hair salon coupons for natural, activity-friendly styles.

Obesity prevention is a particular focus of the sorority's health outreach, because of the high rates among African American women. One program is PALS (Physical Activity Liaison to my Sisters), in which participants attend *Lift Off!* trainings and work to identify "sister" agencies willing to develop and implement fit practice and policy changes.

The project has proven exceptionally popular among members, who complain when the *Lift Off!* somehow gets left off the agenda or bypassed. Several sorors credit *Lift Off!* with sparking their journey back to fitness, boasting that they've lost a little weight and, most importantly, kept it off. And a number of Deltas report having introduced the recess break in their workplace, church, or professional association.

Profile 5. St. John's CME Church, Winston-Salem, NC

St. John's CME (Christian Methodist Episcopal) Church, in Winston Salem, North Carolina, is a typical family-oriented southern church —it offers services throughout the week, lots of good food, and few opportunities for physical activity. That changed in 2005 when the church pastor, Bobby Best, agreed to allow one of his parishioners, my mentee and collaborator Melicia Whitt-Glover, to implement an eight-week physical activity study for the congregation. Although participants did well during the study and increased their activity levels, participants reverted to their usual sedentary behavior when the study was over.

Fast forward to 2007, when a new pastor came on board. Moses Goldmon, with dual roles as a pastor and a faculty member at Shaw University Divinity School, had training in health education and a passion and calling for improving health in congregations. He started by supporting healthier food options at church events and quickly moved to health behaviors, including physical activity, stress management, and regular checkups. Healthy behaviors was a regular topic during his Sunday morning sermons and weekly Bible studies. Pastor Goldmon's research life focused on incorporating one's faith into one's daily lifestyle, including self-care and healthy behaviors. He reinvigorated the church's health ministry and encouraged activities that promoted health in the church.

A 2008 transition supplement from UCLA, awarded by the Robert Wood Johnson Foundation for *Lift Off!/Instant Recess* dissemination, kickstarted the process. St. John's received a $500 mini-grant to disseminate exercise break materials for use in the faith setting. Health ministry leaders in the church decided to use the activity breaks to convince women that they could be physically active. They started by inviting women to gather at the church on Mondays to go through the 10-minute activity break routine. Participants became so excited and enthusiastic that the mini-grant funds were used to pay for a trained exercise instructor to lead group exercises once a week at the church. Classes continued for a year with a dedicated few until mini-grant funds ran out. The church agreed to provide additional funding to continue to support the exercise leader. Seniors in the weekly noontime Bible study expressed interest in participating in exercise classes at the church but mentioned that they did not feel comfortable going out in the evenings. Pastor Goldmon requested that exercise breaks be used at the end of Bible study each week and, to increase participation, he began stopping Bible study 10 minutes early to engage the entire group in exercise (including the pastor).

The minister became so encouraged by the response during Bible study that he requested an activity break during the morning service (during the normal "meet and greet" time). Melicia was nervous about whether people would get up and exercise in their suits and church hats but agreed to try. In March 2010, they implemented the first activity break during service. The response from the congregation was enthusiastic, a pleasant surprise to Melicia. People who had never talked or moved much during service were up in the aisles swinging their arms and exercising! Even the older people who needed assistance to get in and out of the church and who couldn't stand up and participate did what they could by moving their arms while sitting. The pastors stood up in the pulpit and did the break in their robes, backed by the choir (also in their robes). The drummer even joined in and provided an extra beat. They did only 5 minutes of the activity break, but Melicia described the energy for the rest of the service as "so high you could almost reach out and touch it!" After the service, people in the congregation were coming up to her and talking about how much fun they had doing the exercise. Most gratifying for the health ministry was that 10 new people joined the weekly exercise class, several of whom mentioned that they hadn't thought they could exercise, but after the break, felt they could do it.

According to Melicia, it will take quite a rearranging of the church schedule to include an activity break every week (there are usually several special announcements and a fairly packed agenda on Sundays), but the health ministry is working toward making them a more regular offering. People were still talking about the worship service activity break two months later, at the time of this writing, so there's little doubt they'll continue.

Getting leaders to adopt innovations can be challenging, but not as challenging as keeping them going over time. Change is tough, as much so for organizations as for individuals. As these profiles demonstrate, the agencies we've worked with have had varying levels of success, and every change effort is a work in progress. The old song "Everything Must Change" certainly applies here, since at any point in time, circumstances can shift to reinforce these policies and practices—or relegate them to the back burner, hopefully only temporarily.

WRAPPING IT UP AND PUTTING A BOW ON IT

By targeting audiences in organizational settings—work sites, schools, churches, and civic and social groups, *Instant Recess* offers a mechanism for bolstering individual motivation. It can also circumvent economic constraints and cultural norms and values that place a low priority on leisure time physical activity. And it works through social controls (like peer pressure and expectations) and social support and organizational self-interest.

The recess model is an "opt out," or "push," approach. Pushing makes the physically active choice the default choice—difficult to avoid and requiring effort to opt out. Just as sitting on the couch is the easy choice, so these organizational practice and policy change strategies make the active choices the *easy* choices because people have to make a conscious decision *not* to participate each time they're exposed. Simultaneously, the inactive choices are made more difficult. Opting out incurs cost, inconvenience, and social sanctions—disapproval, ridicule, or marginalization.

Prolonged sitting may, in this way, be rendered as socially unacceptable as drinking and driving, or smoking. After all, we wouldn't even *think* of cooping people up for hours at a time during professional meetings or at social gatherings without offering some sort of food and beverage refreshments. That would be considered impolite and unmannerly! Why shouldn't brief recess breaks be included among the socially obligatory "refreshments"? Providing 10 minutes of activity (one-third of the "RDA" for physical activity) is a lot easier and cheaper than offering a nutritious meal—constituting one-third of our daily food needs. It's not the whole answer, but it sure is a step in the right direction!

Typically, work breaks have been reserved for smoking and coffee (health-compromising or health-neutral behaviors), and have been aggressively protected by workers and their unions. Converting or expanding these breaks into opportunities for reducing stress and socializing while improving health capitalizes on the social and physical infrastructure of the workplace. If they can be successfully framed as an entitlement garnering union protection and advocacy, there's a lot of potential to make *Instant Recess* a household name, *and* national pastime.

SIX *Instant Recess*—What's Good for the Waistline Is Good for the Bottom Line!

OK, this is all well and good and warm and fuzzy, but you need something you can hang your hat on if you're going to persuade others to get on board—especially the cynics you're dealing with every day. Perhaps you're convinced by now that activity breaks are manageable, but really, what good are they? What difference do they make, and what kind of proof is there that they work? A lot of things sound good on paper, but how do they translate in practice? What's the longer-term experience of the recess model? Where has this been tried, and what are the hard outcomes? What can you take to the bank?

DOES IT WORK?

There's growing evidence that incorporating brief structured group physical activity breaks into the daily organizational routine, particularly in schools and workplaces, is gaining momentum. Researchers have demonstrated improvements in individual attitudes and medical test results (repetitive motion injuries, bone density), as well as organizational productivity (longer attention spans and fewer visits to the principal's office among students in school, less absenteeism and "presenteeism" at work). In a Los Angeles County Department of Public Health study, we assigned twenty-six regularly scheduled meetings or training seminars to get either a 10-minute exercise break or only the usual phone or bathroom breaks. After participating in the exercise break, sedentary county workers in the experimental group rated their health or fitness status *lower* (and therefore more realistically) than did sedentary individuals in control meetings with no breaks (Yancey, Wold, et al. 2004). This difference in rating did not happen among the more active workers. A common complaint, as always, was "Are you sure it's only been five minutes?" Apparently, getting out of breath after only a few minutes broke through these workers' blissful ignorance, serving as a teachable moment linking their inactivity to their poor health and fitness status.

Here's further evidence for the broad cultural salience of the recess approach. I was attending a board of directors meeting of the Public Health Institute, a large California-based nonprofit, in Puerto Vallarta several winters ago—one of our board members, Dr. Roberto Tapia, was the head of Mexico's Public Health Department at the time. Of course, we've been doing activity breaks at our meetings and retreats for a decade, since I joined the board around the time I was developing the *Lift Off!* intervention at LA County. I was pleasantly surprised when this photo popped up on a slide by one of the presenters, along with some promising preliminary findings from an intervention similar to ours with 335 mostly overweight or obese employees at the Mexican Ministry of Health in Mexico City. After a year of *Pausa para tu Salud* (Pause for Your Health), employees lost about two pounds on average and reduced their waist measurements by more than half an inch. So we teamed up with Roberto and his colleagues (Lara et al. 2008) to further analyze and publish this data. I consider the *Pausa* findings particularly compelling because the data did not come from study volunteers (who are quite different from

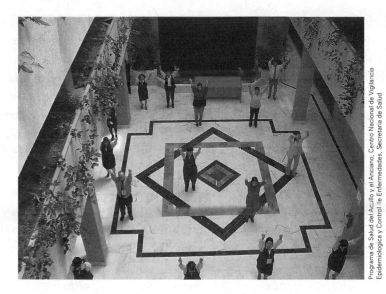

Figure 16. Pausa para tu Salud (Pause for Your Health), a daily office-wide activity break at the Mexican Ministry of Health, Mexico City. The weight and "waist" loss outcomes were compelling because these were regular folks, not study volunteers.

normal folks, who are highly unlikely to tolerate being poked, prodded, and made to fill out long survey forms unless there's something wrong with them). Rather, we analyzed existing data from clinical exams done annually on all employees and, at the one-year follow-up, had data on 75 percent of those for whom we had baseline data. That's a much lower attrition rate than for most work-site studies and makes me more confident that the results can be replicated in other places.

Since the recess model originated in schools at the same time it did in the workplace, it's not surprising that integrating activity breaks would flourish in that milieu, especially in challenging circumstances—overcrowding, cuts in PE and recess time, and disciplinary and attention problems. In fact, most of the studies of structuring brief bouts of activity into daily routine have involved schools. There are excellent evaluations of these breaks demonstrating their contribution to both health and learning, including *Take 10!*—the one that Bill Kohl developed around the same time as our *Lift Off!*—*Energizers, Making the Grade with Diet and Exercise,* and *PASS & CATCH.* The delivery system for these interventions is generally different from that of *Instant Recess,* requiring that teachers work the activity into their lesson plans as they prepare for class or that they lead the activity themselves, or both. *Instant Recess,* on the other hand, is "plug and play"—technology mediated, music driven, and intended as a mental respite for students and teachers. However, the endpoint in both cases is physical activity participation, so the outcomes of these studies are applicable to the recess model.

Physical Activity Across the Curriculum (PAAC), a federally funded University of Kansas study of a variation of *Take 10!,* successfully engaged 60 to 80 percent of elementary school non-PE teachers in conducting 10-minute exercise breaks in twenty-four public schools in three eastern Kansas cities: Kansas City, Topeka, and Lawrence (Gibson et al. 2008; Honas et al. 2008; Donnelly et al. 2009). While *Take 10!* emphasizes being active while learning, PAAC focuses on making the activity integral to the lesson. Study staff provided teacher training in one six-hour, off-site in-service session at the beginning of each school year. Interestingly, from the standpoint of *Instant Recess*'s innovation, music to use in leading the exercise sessions was one of the most frequent requests in the staff training sessions—they began distributing oldies CDs popular with both teachers and students. The gradual increase in the number of teachers engaged each year and number of minutes provided reflected a progressive cultural norm change (an average of 70 minutes a week of activity, and nearly 50 percent of teachers achieving the goal of 90 to 100 minutes a week after two years). The PAAC increased the kids' physical activity levels, in school and outside school—on both weekdays and weekends. This finding is particularly significant because, like other recent evidence (Lynch, Corbin, and Sidman 2009), it contradicts the concept of "compensation": some have argued that restricted activity during the school day because of less recess and PE may be offset by compensatory increases outside school. The converse is that adding structured physical activity may lead to decreases in other venues, but that's not consistent with the PAAC data.

PAAC also improved academic achievement in terms of reading, math, spelling, and composition scores. When the investigators looked specifically at the nine of fourteen intervention schools that averaged more than 75 minutes of active lessons weekly, students gained less weight than those in control schools. Not surprisingly, when teachers were active with the students, student physical activity levels were significantly higher. Earlier studies of *Take 10!* have also demonstrated the feasibility and utility of this approach in regularly engaging students and teachers in exercise of sufficient intensity and duration to count toward the total recommended by the Centers for Disease Control and Prevention. For example, James Stewart and his colleagues (2004) found that third through fifth graders burned 27 to 36 kilocalories and racked up step counts of eight hundred to a thousand with each break.

Given the incursion of sedentariness and obesity into younger and younger age groups, the *Take 10!* folks have developed Animal Trackers, an adaptation of their active lessons for preschoolers (Williams et al. 2009). They recently published process data from a pilot test of the intervention at Head Start sites in New Mexico, showing that they were able to deliver an average of 47 additional minutes of structured physical activity per week (4.1 sessions per week averaging 11.4 minutes per session).

Energizer activity breaks (Mahar et al. 2006) along the lines of *Take 10!* used grade-appropriate learning materials, involved no equipment, and required little teacher training (one 45-minute training session). Not only were kids more active during the school day, but on-task behavior improved by 8 percent overall after the *Energizer* breaks and by 20 percent among the least on-task students (those who were on-task less than 50 percent of the time before *Energizers* were instituted).

A different model from *Take 10!* of delivering activity breaks involved three basic school environmental changes: (1) restructuring the school day to provide 15 minutes of teacher-led activity each morning to start the day, (2) access to a free breakfast program for all students to promote nutritionally sound practices, and (3) a reversal of the order of lunch and recess. The last strategy, *Recess Before Lunch*, was developed to capitalize on the body's craving for water after exertion—studies have found less "plate waste," especially of fruits and veggies, when kids eat after moving and sweating than before. Adopting these three changes produced a 67 percent decline in nurse visits, a 58 percent decrease in disciplinary referrals, and an increase in academic performance such that the school improved from passing two of the state achievement tests to passing all five after four years (Sibley et al. 2008).

PASS & CATCH is yet another school model. Coordinated Approach to Child Health (*CATCH*) is one of the pioneering activity-focused physical education upgrades as a part of a schoolwide environmental change approach. *PASS & CATCH* adds brief and enjoyable activity breaks folded into the in-class didactic curriculum that has been found to improve math scores for all third and fourth graders and to improve both reading and math scores for poorly adapting students (Murray 2009).

On our UCLA Kaiser Permanente Center for Health Equity Web site, we regularly update an annotated bibliography of all of the articles addressing the feasibility, effectiveness, and dissemination capacity of brief bouts of physical activity incorporated into the routine of various organizations all over the world. This burgeoning literature speaks to the universality and practicality of the approach.

DISSEMINATION

Our Experience

Considerable diffusion of the recess model has already occurred in Los Angeles and elsewhere, with no more investment in marketing than my lectures and seminars incorporating these breaks. For example, at a 2006 community cancer prevention seminar funded by the Centers for Disease Control and Prevention, attended by about 350 representatives of 200 Southern California health and social services agencies, at least two-thirds responded to a request for a show of hands indicating they had participated in exercise breaks during organizational meetings or events. A number of our collaborators have begun to adopt and adapt the recess break concept into their own research. Wendell Taylor at the University of Texas has named them "booster breaks," securing a small federal agency grant to evaluate their efficacy.

In 2008–09, we subcontracted a Robert Wood Johnson Foundation Active Living Research dissemination award to Wake Forest University to provide $500 mini-grants, training, and technical assistance to ten churches and schools willing to adopt *Lift Off!* for three months. (One was St. John's CME Church, profiled in the previous chapter.) Preliminary findings on about two hundred people revealed increases in physical activity—self-reported and objectively monitored by accelerometer (a glorified step counter)—and decreases in blood pressure and weight, such that many people moved down from the obese to the overweight category.

At Union Chapel Baptist Church, one of the participating churches, the Rev. Konnie Robinson had been conscientious about his flock's health. The congregation included several nurses, and the ministry had begun some sporadic health promotion efforts such as health fairs and identifying healthier meal options. But they came on board immediately when they heard about the *Instant Recess* model. The Rev. Robinson set the policy that any activity at the church lasting 30 minutes or longer would include 10 minutes of physical activity. While the minimum number of people who had to agree to be weighed and measured at baseline for the church to qualify for the study was twenty, fifty signed up at Union Chapel. And they participated in recess breaks religiously—during choir rehearsals, deaconness and missionary meetings, Bible study, Sunday School, and yes, even during the regular Sunday morning service. The pastor introduced activity into the "meet and greet" portion of the program, and the organist would push the tempo and the congregation would get to movin' around. It startled some of the visitors to the church who hadn't been introduced to this particular form of worship! He even took it upon himself to introduce activity breaks when he spoke at church conventions, often to crowds 250 or more.

Deltra Bonner, who heads the health and human services ministry for Union Chapel, was particularly animated about the experience. Deltra found that the practice really "took" among the seniors and the middle-aged women—those of us, as she described, whose "hourglass figures were a thing of the past," but who hadn't quite given up the ghost on maintaining their looks. As people started losing a few pounds, they got a lot of encouragement from others, and that social support and interaction made a big difference, from Deltra's perspective. She attributed the successful institutionalization of the exercise break to three elements: committed, boisterous ministerial leadership by example; an implementation infrastructure—in this case, the health ministry—to take responsibility for establishing and maintaining momentum and to be accountable to the pastor; and individual members of the congregation taking ownership and bringing their own skills and resources to the table to make participation fun and stimulating. And for some, activity definitely spilled over from the short breaks to longer periods of engagement. For example, one member's husband was a football coach at a local university. He was pressed into service to run a three-session "boot camp." The Wednesday evening Bible study group began meeting an hour earlier for a walk. Deltra admitted that they don't lift off quite as often after the first year as they did in the beginning, but she was adamant that it still happened regularly—especially when the Rev. Robinson's around. A recent development really sealing the deal on Union Chapel's fitness commitment was a letter of appreciation from President Obama for holding him and his family in prayer during the early-morning prayer walks.

The Centers for Disease Control and Prevention has also bought into the promise of the recess model to get America moving, with a $4.25 million grant for a Center of Excellence in the Elimination of Disparities at UCLA to disseminate this intervention approach. This grant has supported our center's most significant policy success to date—formal adoption of a daily *Lift Off!* on paid time by the Orange County Health Care Agency (more about this later).

Our research team also received a renewal of our CDC Cancer Prevention and Control Research Network grant. The original grant, spearheaded by my close colleague Dr. Roshan Bastani, helped to establish a critical mass of researchers in our division at the cancer center working on physical activity and nutrition. The new grant is helping us break new ground in cultural adaptation of the recess model. For example, we just collaborated with Montana State University, documentary filmmakers Story Road Films, Cascade County, and the Sioux and Assiniboine

Indian tribes of Montana's Fort Peck Reservation to produce *Moving with Tradition,* a powwow-dance-inspired *Instant Recess* break—including shots of tribal leaders exercising at a tribal council meeting.

Another vote of confidence came from the National Institutes of Health, which has funded a follow-on study to our pilot work site wellness investigation of this approach in twenty-five Southern California human services agencies (several of which were profiled in chapter 5), one that will test the model in seventy-five to eighty new sites. We also got a fair amount of national media attention in 2009 (including NPR and ESPN stories archived on their Web sites).

Business Case

OK. So we've got people on board in nonprofits, churches, and government. What about corporate America? You can have all of the scientific evidence in the world that it's healthier, but companies won't institute *Instant Recess* unless you can show it'll improve their bottom line.

Recess for adults in the workplace may sound like a radical, anticorporate idea, but workers and managers cotton to it immediately once it's explained. Restricting vending machine offerings to nutrient-rich foods or making nutrient-poor foods less accessible can smack of the nanny state to some. Recess, on the other hand, may be sold as a benefit for workers. And it is exactly that—it's an energy boost, stress release, and mood lift. So yes, it's radical, inasmuch as it departs from the norm. But *Instant Recess* can help a company's bottom line, while, umm, reducing its employees' bottom lines, if you get my drift.

The levers to encourage *Instant Recess* differ between public and nonprofit agencies and private sector organizations. In the former, it's more about mission—the responsibility for the residents they serve, with particular sensitivity to social and health inequities. However, all organizations are employers, even in those industries whose products are a big part of the problem. In both sectors, there's a major push toward increasing productivity, whatever the deliverables, and containing health-related costs.

Some industries can even reap direct savings if the entire US popu-

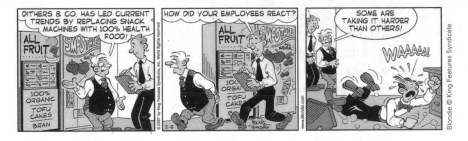

Figure 17.   Some can be a bit resistant to change!

lation becomes more fit. The airline industry's getting killed by fuel consumption costs, worse since they've had to increase the average estimated weight per passenger from 150 to 180 pounds. (And that was a few years ago—imagine what it is now!) The sedentariness of their customers while on the plane is a health hazard and a corporate liability. A variation of *Instant Recess* on airline rides could be an immediate benefit to the bottom line and a boon to dissemination. It'd be great exposure for the program among a huge captive audience of leaders and decision makers racking up frequent-flier miles, and activity breaks could reduce the risk of blood clots in the legs and lungs of seniors and even heavy younger people. Managed care organizations are another prime example. Stronger and lighter-weight patients would not only demand less care and consume fewer resources but also throw out fewer backs of the nursing staff trying to lift them!

If managers and executives try to argue that they can't afford to give workers a break for exercise, the experience of L.L. Bean, based in Portland, Maine, seems to show they can't afford not to. For two decades, L.L. Bean has been stopping its assembly lines three times a day for 5-minute stretch breaks, and reports that the increase in productivity more than makes up for the activity time. The company gets a 100 percent return on investment, or 30 minutes of output measured in bags, belts, and boxers in exchange for those 15 minutes (California Nutrition Network and California Department of Health Service 2004). The employees reduced their work-related injuries from fourteen per year to essentially none within the first three years after implementing the breaks. Lately, they've even begun doing a few minutes each hour.

When I interviewed her for this book, Susan Tufts, the company's wellness manager, equated these breaks to other commonplace occupational safety and health practices, like asking someone to wear safety glasses if the work is potentially hazardous to the eyes (Simon 2006).

Susan emphasized that the company began to develop a culture of wellness in 1982, seven years before she instituted the exercise breaks. This reflected the vision of Leon Gorman, the grandson of Bean's founder, now in his seventies, who still chairs the board of directors. The initial changes included fully equipped and staffed exercise rooms in each of their thirteen work units, completion of health risk assessments tied to the company benefits package with monetary incentives, individual risk-reduction counseling, and nutrition and cooking classes. They've had some major successes, such as reducing their employee smoking rates from 25 percent in 1985 (the same as the population of their Portland location) to 9 percent (compared with a 21 to 22 percent statewide smoking rate). However, she acknowledged that only about 25 percent of employees take advantage of their voluntary workout opportunities. The exercise breaks have been the cornerstone of the cultural change because they're the only way to reach the majority of the employee population.

Nor are people especially likely to exercise on their own even when encouraged to do so during break time carved out for that purpose. In a study of Internal Revenue Service data entry operators, Traci Galinsky and her colleagues (2007) found that only 25 percent of those instructed to do 2-minute stretching routines during break time reported actually doing so during the conventional break schedule (two 15-minute breaks per day) and only 39 percent did so when four additional 5-minute supplemental breaks were added. Those who received the four supplemental daily breaks reported less musculoskeletal discomfort and fewer eyestrain symptoms than those on the conventional two-break schedule. The mean rate of data entry of the operators participating in the supplementary breaks was also higher by more than 250 keystrokes per hour, such that the total number of documents they entered per day was comparable to those of employees on the conventional schedule, despite their being logged on to their computers for 19 fewer minutes on average. Only half of those in each group were instructed to exercise, and there were no differences between those in the "stretching" and "no stretching" groups in each study arm. However, most people reported walking for at least some portion of each break, and the sample size of 51 workers was too small after being divided into the four different conditions (conventional stretching, conventional no stretching, supplementary stretching, and supplementary no stretching) to detect the minor differences in physical activity participation between these groups. Clearly a culture of moving around during breaks had been established and likely contributed to the positive outcomes demonstrated.

Another example of structuring in activity is provided by Replacements, a 550-employee Fortune 500 distributor of china, crystal, and silver. Based in Greensboro, North Carolina, Replacements has successfully improved workplace safety since instituting 10-minute group stretch breaks on the clock every morning and afternoon about five years ago. Two-thirds of its staff work in a warehouse, half are women, most are American-born whites, though a sizable number of the whites are Eastern European refugees, and a quarter are of color, mostly black with some South American Latinos. Replacement's contract occupational nurse had identified two departments with large numbers of musculoskeletal complaints. She introduced the stretches to one department on an instruction sheet for individual use at their desks. In the other department, she turned on the music and employees did the stretches as a group "on the clock." Both departments had fewer doctor-treated musculoskeletal disorders. However, the number and severity of musculoskeletal complaints declined significantly only in the latter department. This was probably because, as Galinsky and her colleagues (ibid.) documented, the stretches got done more often by most of the employees rather than the select few that typically participate on a self-initiated voluntary basis—duhhh! The breaks were scheduled into the daily routine, and employees enjoyed doing them. They found them relaxing, energizing, and socially engaging. Since that time, the company's experience modification rate, a government indicator that compares the number, severity, and frequency of workers' comp claims across work sites, has gone down every year. This has translated into savings for the company through decreased workers' comp insurance premiums at the time of each annual renewal.

As is always the case, leadership is a necessary ingredient in creating a culture of wellness permeating the entire organization. The founder of Replacements sparks competition among the senior staff, along with departmental performance measures, on blood pressure and cholesterol levels. He rents stretch limos to take female employees of all positions within the organization in shifts to get annual mammograms. The company also has a 17 percent utilization rate of their employee assistance program, compared with the 2 percent considered a good showing industry-wide. Most of the staff completes health risk assessments, with nearly 20 percent enrolled in disease management.

I can attest to this myself, up close and personal, from my special sample of one, namely my assistant and Head Diva in Charge, Danielle Osby. She's been working for me for ten years, first with Los Angeles County Division of Chronic Disease Prevention and Health Promotion and, since 2001, at UCLA. Danielle's got a cesspool of a family history, metabolically speaking. Her mom had gastric bypass surgery before age fifty-five, with poorly controlled diabetes and hypertension as the precipitating factors, and diabetes complications killed her dad before he was fifty! No member of her family had kept her uterus after age forty. Yet, as a 5-foot-10-inch Amazonian woman somewhere north of the cutoff for obesity, she hasn't gained a pound during this decade (and has shed some in the past few years), leads exercise breaks without a hint of breathlessness (you can see for yourself in our first *Lift Off!* DVD), helps choreograph recess breaks, and pushing forty now, still has her uterus and not even borderline hypertension or pre-diabetes. Danielle and her family chalk this up to the culture of wellness we have created in our workplace, because her cousins and other relatives in her age cohort are gaining more weight and are being diagnosed with chronic diseases at an earlier age than their parents. That's typical of the aging and secular trends of weight and waist gain, and earlier and earlier sickness and disability sweeping the country. In our office, we're serious about walking the talk, and our goal from the inception of our push organizational policy and practice change efforts has been preventing weight gain and deferring obesity and chronic disease co-morbidities, not trying to make everyone into skinny Minnies.

Another corporate model aligning injury prevention and fitness promotion comes from the Westinghouse electronic assembly plant in College Station, Texas. A group of employees who assembled computer boards there was randomly assigned to perform a set of twenty-three flexibility and strength exercises, designed to prevent lower-back and carpal tunnel injury, for 10 minutes each day on company time under supervision. Daily participation rates were between 97 and 100 percent. Six months later, significant improvements were observed in wrist flexion, wrist extension, lower-back flexibility, fatigue, and mood, compared with results from a control group that did not participate in these exercises (Pronk et al. 1995).

Johnson & Johnson has been a pioneer in work-site wellness, beginning in the 1970s with its *Live for Life* program. Because J&J encompasses 250 separate companies on several continents, it sets goals and influences the culture, but does not prescribe exactly how component agencies attain their objectives. Many choose the usual—on-site fitness facilities, step contests, and individual coaching and counseling. But several strategies are also utilized across the corporation that structure physical activity into the workday, including a pilot project to equip workstations with low-speed treadmills. And in "Walk with the Doctor," company physicians lead 10-minute walks on paid time with co-workers gathered along the way. Ergonomic stretch breaks are common push strategies in jobs in which workers are prone to musculoskeletal injury. One J&J company, Cordis, with manufacturing plants in such locales as Miami Lakes, Florida, and Juarez, Mexico, has taken this to another level reminiscent of *Recess*. It pipes music onto the shop floor, and workers engage in short dance breaks they call Bidi Bidi Bom Bom. Beyond the benefits to individual employee health, these breaks are associated with lower rates of injury and, at least anecdotally, enhanced productivity. In an interview for this book, Dr. Fik Isaac, J&J's executive director of worldwide health and safety technical services, echoed the sentiments of most, that leadership is the key factor in establishing a corporate culture of wellness. And though the independent contribution of activity integral to organizational routine cannot be assessed, the aggregate is working. Between the baseline data collection years of 1995–2000 just prior to the rollout of a J&J "Move and Make It Matter" physical activity campaign, and the 2007–08 follow-up, the proportion of employees who reported being physically inactive dropped 20 percent, from 39 percent to 31 percent.

It's hard to determine the true amount of activity that people engage in from what they report themselves. When monitored by accelerometers secured to their waists, adults engage in only 6 to 10 minutes of moderate to vigorous physical activity per day, but they report twice that much on public health surveillance surveys. This suggests that participation in a single 10-minute activity bout each day could more than double the average US physical activity level. If the direct health care costs of physical inactivity are $128 to $330 per person yearly (Andreyeva and Sturm 2006, Dull et al. 2003), and this practice change moved just 10 percent of the workforce out of the sedentary category (those who exercise less than 10 minutes a week), the annual savings could easily surpass $1 billion in avoided hospital, pharmaceutical, physician, and other medical costs alone. Commensurate savings resulting from improved worker productivity, lower workers' comp claims, and decreased absenteeism and leave could magnify considerably the savings from direct health care costs.

Cost is undoubtedly a key constraint in a corporation's willingness to implement a new approach. The level of risk reduction needed to offset the costs of comprehensive wellness programs is considered to be modest. The higher the proportion of the total employee population engaged (because those with more room for improvement are involved), the lower the intervention effectiveness can be while still remaining at least cost neutral. Unlike comprehensive efforts, however, the ongoing cost to implement activity breaks is negligible—very modest amounts of employee time to participate, coordination time (from a single staff member or an employee wellness or health and safety advisory committee) and, perhaps, incentives like pedometers or comp time. Start-up costs are also quite modest—materials purchase (CDs, DVDs, instructional cards, and brochures) and coordinator (program champion) time for training and support.

Previous workplace wellness efforts involving only "pull" strategies such as gyms, stair prompts, stairwell improvements, showers, and bike racks along with lunchtime walking groups or workouts have rarely delivered such substantial returns on investment. That's because only the diehards stick to it after the initial excitement wears off. And since most of them use their own discretionary time and money for active recreation anyway, there's limited additional benefit to be gained. In other words, without the organizational buy-in to encourage activity during nondiscretionary work hours (company time), regular partici- pants, over time, will primarily be leaner, more active, and healthier than most workers. This only shifts their activity from their own leisure time to work time, resulting in no widespread changes, fewer individual improvements, and few if any organizational benefits. The effects of adding 10 minutes per day to the activity levels of people who already exercise are less substantive.

On the other hand, adding 10 minutes of exercise to the daily rou- tines of sedentary individuals might represent a 300 percent increase in energy expenditure (and at least a 100 percent increase for the average person), with the potential to stabilize weight and waist measurements! Push interventions—like scheduled group exercise breaks, walking meetings, and parking and elevator restrictions—that rely *less* on indi- vidual initiative and motivation to be active (examples provided earlier in table 1), may have greater organizational and societal impact, such as increased business productivity and medical care cost savings, than past efforts focused on pull strategies. This is particularly true in ethnically diverse populations.

There's certainly been quite a bit of progress, mostly in the private sector, in advancing push changes to the built environment. Our team at UCLA conducted a pilot project at the downtown Los Angeles Caltrans headquarters building with an innovative architectural design with skip- stop elevators (nondisabled employees can enter or exit on floors 1, 4, 7, or 11) and appealing open stairwells nested into the work spaces with ambient light streaming in. At the suburban headquarters for Capital One in my old haunt, Richmond, Virginia, architects strategically placed the food court at the end of a string of buildings, rather than more cen- trally, to encourage utilitarian walking (Zernike 2003). That particular strategy may actually be a two-fer—people that don't want to make the walk may eat less often or may bring their meals from home, which are usually more nutritious. Of course, if they permit the installation in each building of vending machines offering highly processed snack foods or beverages, that'll kinda defeat the purpose. The same architectural firm also designed the Sprint campus in a suburb of my hometown, Kansas City, Kansas. Sprint banished all parking garages to the periphery of the office park, prompting employees to walk as far as a half mile between buildings. Similarly, its wide windowed staircases are faster and more convenient than the hydraulic (slowed) elevators. I've also seen photos of Fortune 500 corporate board rooms tricked out with elliptical cross-trainers and treadmills around the tables instead of chairs.

At first, Sprint provided trolleys, though walking was usually faster. So the active choice wasn't mandatory, but it was a whole lot easier and more convenient—in other words, the path of least resistance. Despite their initial trepidation, many of the mouse potatoes acclimated nicely to the "forced wellness program" and have been pleasantly surprised by actually enjoying the walk. After the first year, the demand for the trolley fell so precipitously that the company just dropped it. Of course, that's not to say that some folks aren't still spending a lot of time circling the parking lot in hopes of finding a closer spot (ibid.). But notice that in all of the examples I've mentioned, the primary beneficiaries are largely affluent men.

My recess model emphasizes organizational practice and policy change push strategies because they favor population segments that are more sedentary—women, people of color, low-income groups. These are the groups that are more inclined to prefer structured group activities like dance, and that typically have many barriers—like high crime, a lack of parks or gyms, and no sidewalks—to active leisure or human-fueled transport. As I've stressed throughout the book, to make a population-wide dent, the bulk of our intervention approach must preferentially influence these segments because the small amounts of activity in terms of intensity and duration induced by most environmental changes will have the greatest societal impact on those at higher risk for the chronic diseases associated with a sedentary lifestyle.

I've recently run across several more great applications of the recess model. I met Dean Orion, a writer-producer who heads a start-up company called Minds at Play, at a childhood obesity conference in LA. When he worked for Imagineering at Disney World in Florida several years ago, one of his tasks was to develop "queue-line interactive entertainment" to help quell customer boredom and unrest during the long waits, sometimes upward of two hours, for popular rides. He and his team created a number of four- to five-minute DVD virtual worlds with which people could interact by moving their bodies in various ways. Mounted cameras and five screens were each capable of capturing the movements of about fifty people. Interestingly, the crowds consistently performed additional unexpected movements beyond those that controlled the avatars, and these spread from one small group (like a family) to the next. For instance, people flapped their arms to direct the movement of a large bird when only leaning from side to side actually moved the bird. The intervention seemed to have succeeded on several levels. The number of park visitors who rated the Soarin' ride "excellent" more than doubled, from 18 to 40 percent, after Disney started the interactive entertainment. And the surveys didn't ask about the waiting-line videos—the experience influenced the rating of the ride itself, which hadn't changed.

Another example came across the newswires last year in the wake of pop star Michael Jackson's death. A security consultant for the Cebu provincial government in the Philippines, Byron Garcia, started a compulsory fitness regimen for prison inmates consisting of marching to pop music in a bid to increase participation in exercises. The Filipino prisoner "Thriller" breaks (a well-choreographed, 15-minute routine to music from Michael Jackson's 1980s bestselling album) have been featured on YouTube and generated millions of views. They have dramatically improved discipline, according to Garcia, quelling discontent and reducing violence. While no one's forced to exercise, high rates of participation are generated by the threat of the withdrawal of conjugal visits and other coveted privileges. Garcia's been taken aback by the worldwide popularity of the video clips, which he'd originally posted solely for the purpose of sharing his work with others in the penal community (BBC News 2009).

No less compelling is the approach of a Buffalo, New York, exercise physiologist Dan Mitchell, who contacted me after our UCLA *Instant Recess* breaks were featured on NPR. Dan's company, the Soap Box, contracts with businesses nationally to empower employees and cultivate creativity in the workplace by introducing 3- to 5-minute exercise time blocks. His perspective is that people rarely innovate from a position of comfort. In fact, his clients find that mild to moderate discomfort is almost required for the creative process to really kick in. So he induces this level of "controlled discomfort" with exercise, in a safe and positive way. Dan changes the "result expectation" of exercise to production instead of the usual emphasis on physical image. Since most of us are our own worst critics, this perspective can be freeing for many, along with the sense of accomplishment and gratification from mastering the movements over time with practice. Dan's a black belt in aikido, so the movements he's created are based on martial arts, which probably enhances the "out of body" nature of the experience for his clients. He has lots of satisfied customers to show for his efforts—they report improvements in both the volume and quality of creative output. Not to mention boosts in confidence and initiative: some have been moved to go out and host their first independent art shows or record their first pieces of music.

All in all, the recess model is as consistent with American values as apple pie—with only half a scoop of ice cream, please. First, it stresses independence, entrepreneurialism, competition, and self-regulation. And it's democratic: everyone can participate with whatever resources are available.

Second, you get a robust multiplier effect within and between organizations in various sectors, spurred by leadership commitment and engagement *and* by grassroots or frontline empowerment, ownership, and entitlement. In most settings, the "bottom up" swaying of colleagues and co-workers with persistence and support is just as critical to success as "top down" economic arguments of increases in efficiency and lower health care costs.

Third, the opportunity to change organizational practices and policies is immediate, especially for decision makers and high-profile individuals. The charge is to "look in the mirror" and take immediate action. So often you leave a meeting, lecture, or rally hyped up and ready to crush the opposition and conquer the problem. But the energy dissipates if there's nothing you can *do* right away and the priorities in your life reassert themselves and reclaim your full attention. Also, many if not most approaches to increasing physical activity are focused on children and child-serving settings. That focus engenders complacency on the part of those not professionally responsible for children. For instance, despite children's exposure to secondhand smoke creating a rallying cry for early tobacco-control efforts, smoking bans were implemented in a variety of settings not limited to schools and parks. In fact, smoking bans became a core strategy in setting the wheels of change in motion that folks across many societal sectors could either implement or advocate for in their own spheres of influence. This was essential in creating a critical mass of support for tobacco control.

Fourth, the most effective physical activity interventions involve *monitored* activity doses, and those that are palatable to sedentary people. The recess model encompasses both characteristics.

INTERVENTION SPOTLIGHT

I'm presenting here the recess model of the structured group exercise breaks I developed, *Lift Off! LA* and *Instant Recess*, as the major case study. Additional case studies illustrating a range of innovations and adaptations of activity breaks were described in chapter 5 and will be presented later in this chapter.

Original Prototype: Lift Off! LA

The *Lift Off!* break consists of a series of basic aerobic dance, calisthenics, and sports movements with funny and self-explanatory titles, like the Hulk, the Hallelujah, and the Knee High. Simple, moderate-intensity, low-impact moves—aerobic, stretching, and resistance—are performed in 10-minute bouts to music one or more times a day at work or in other organizational settings. *Lift Off!*s have been medically designed for sedentary, overweight, or less fit youth and adults in ordinary street attire. The 10-minute duration reflects the minimum amount of physical activity required to count toward the CDC's 30-minute minimum daily recommendation. I call it the recommended daily allowance, or RDA, a term

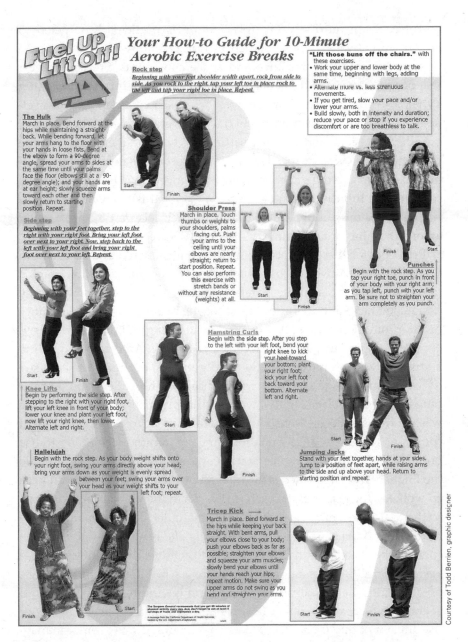

Figure 18. Posters for schools and workplaces featuring real people in street clothes may motivate and remind people how easy it is to do the basic moves—so all it takes is an iPod and 10 minutes!

borrowed from nutrition. The intervention is particularly targeted to largely unmotivated captive audiences (rather than willing volunteers) in environments with resource and space constraints. Studies suggest that people experience immediate benefits in terms of improved meeting dynamics, productivity, feelings of well-being, self-confidence, skill development, and positive reinforcement that motivate them to be more active on other occasions and in other settings. While these exercises can be performed individually, social interaction in groups is necessary to maximize personal and organizational return on investment (see the previous section for a full discussion of the rationale for this). Obviously, people willing to exercise on their own or during their leisure time are usually among the slim minority already meeting CDC recommendations.

Protocols for these exercise breaks were formalized and recorded in English- and Spanish-language videotape, audiotape, and holographic mouse pad materials. These materials and protocols were then used by designated facilitators, who, prior to training by our Los Angeles County health promotion staff, had no professional background in exercise science. Materials were culturally targeted to African American and Latino audiences through music selection and graphics, but reflected inclusivity by featuring video subjects representing both genders and a broad range in ethnicity, age, agility, weight, and physical limitations. Music was commissioned or licensed for a nominal fee from an independent composer for ease of dissemination, since obtaining permission to use popular nationally distributed songs can be difficult and costly. While the English-language video is introduced by me playing basketball with co-workers, the leader of the exercise breaks in the video is my administrative assistant, a mature, overweight, nonathletic black woman. County health promotion staff then trained nursing and health education staff to conduct these breaks and to train others to conduct them, utilizing these *Fuel Up/Lift Off! LA* materials. These breaks proliferated in meetings, presentations, health fair appearances, and community gatherings and events in which county public health staff participated, particularly after the director of public health circulated a memorandum to senior managers encouraging them to take part. As new breaks were choreographed by others on my staff, the litmus test for simplicity was my being able to follow and remember the moves, because my physical talents do not include dance!

The *Lift Off!* was designed to be built into the organizational routine, that is, conducted at a scheduled time of day or implemented during regular meetings, class sessions, or other group activities, and not relegated to discretionary time. As a physicist once said, an object at rest will stay at rest—unless the boss tells him to move his buns. This ensures the participation of many people unlikely to choose activity over sedentary options.

The other "insurance" that these breaks stay focused on the crowd unsold on exercise is a set of specifications we developed over the course of the first year:

- A moderate-intensity pace (a music selection of around 100 to 120 beats per minute)
- Modeling of low-impact or less vigorous modifications of any aggressive or vigorous and high-impact movements such as those aimed at youth
- Attention to neck and lower-back protection, for instance, bending from the hip, not the waist, and keeping the knees behind the plane of the toes
- Inclusion of both aerobic exercise and elements that improve strength or flexibility
- An initial focus on lower-body movements, then adding upper-body movements, to increase energy expenditure and to aid less coordinated individuals in learning the moves
- Simple, easy-to-learn movements for rhythmically challenged, less coordinated, less athletic, or less agile individuals

REACH 2010 and Steppin' Up to Better Health: Instant Recess's *Baby Steps*

The chronic disease division I headed at the Los Angeles County Health Department teamed with a local health advocacy nonprofit to secure funding for "organizational wellness" from the CDC's REACH (Racial and Ethnic Approaches to Community Health) 2010 initiative. Community-based, mainly public and private/nonprofit sector health and human services agencies serving targeted areas of Los Angeles participated in one or more interventions we originally developed at the county to incorporate physical activity into routine organizational practice. These interventions focused on cultivating leadership and establishing policies to model and support activity. Data that we collected on the staff of the participating agencies showed that we'd found a high-risk group of people in need of this type of health promotion: 66 pecent overweight and 30 percent obese; more than 40 percent completely sedentary (less than 10 minutes of physical activity *weekly*); 33 percent with high blood pressure and 26 percent with high cholesterol levels; 86 percent female, 73 percent African American, and 22 percent college educated. We evaluated the project by assessing the extent of the organizational commitment associated with each intervention: participation in exercise breaks at REACH meetings and events (lowest level); inviting REACH staff to lead exercise breaks at organizational functions (low-intermediate level); hosting an organizational wellness training series on practical strategies to increase physical activity and access to healthy food (high-intermediate level); and subcontracting with REACH to provide or expand physical-activity-related programs and services (high level). Nearly half of the approximately 240 participating organizations actively embraced physical activity integration (at the intermediate level or higher), with more than a quarter committed at the highest level of support. This project demonstrated that there was not only need for these services but also broad capacity and support for the organizational integration of physical activity, with the level of commitment varying by type of organization (Yancey, Lewis, et al. 2004).

A total of thirty-five work sites were committed at the high-intermediate level, involving our delivering training in incorporating physical activity and healthy food choices into the routine conduct of business. More than seven hundred individuals who were staff, members, or clients completed the twelve-week curriculum or a shortened and retooled activity break–focused six-week curriculum. Attendance and retention rates between the baseline and follow-up assessment were quite low for the twelve-week curriculum (37 percent showed up for data collection immediately following the last training session). However, attendance rates rebounded to 66 percent for the six-week offering, with 92 percent retention. Feelings of sadness or depression decreased significantly among twelve-week participants, fruit and veggie intake increased significantly (by more than a half serving per day), and BMI decreased marginally, with no significant changes in these outcomes in the six-week group. However, the number of days on which individuals participated in vigorous physical activity increased significantly among six-week participants but not the twelve-week group (Yancey, Lewis, et al. 2006).

WORKING: A Rigorous Federally Funded Test of the Recess Model

In 2005, our UCLA research team received a grant from the National Institutes of Health to formally and rigorously test the recess model, through a work-site intervention, WORKING (Working Out Regularly Keeps Individuals Nurtured and Going—the acronym was coined by one of our community partners). The first phase was a two-year consensus-building process. We engaged 188 individuals representing 59 human services agencies in identifying the set of feasible and potentially effective organizational change strategies to be tested. These policy and practice changes included 10-minute structured group exercise breaks in meetings and at a scheduled time of day as the centerpiece strategy; walking meetings; meetings held at a short distance from attendees' work spaces; healthy refreshments at meetings; healthy (nutrient-rich) foods among vending machine and vendor selections; bowls of fruit or small packages of dried fruit or nuts instead of cookie and candy jars on leaders' desks; healthy food procurement policies for catering and conference facility menus; fund-raising restrictions; and job descriptions of senior manager and line or administrative staff that incorporated wellness policy implementation duties.

The second phase was the pilot-testing of these strategies, which we conducted in twenty-five sites with nearly four hundred employees. We checked their blood pressure, measured their waists, and weighed them at baseline and then six months later, after implementing the strategies. Participants were, on average, female, African American or Latino, middle-aged, well-educated (66 percent had at least some college), obese, and relatively sedentary (fewer than 15 percent reported moderate physical activity on five or more days a week). Average TV viewing was more than two hours each weekday and nearly three and a half hours on weekend days. Forty percent had drunk at least one nondiet soda during the past twenty-four hours, and a third consumed fruits, vegetables, or whole grains less than three days per week.

Organizations, 96 percent of which were public or private health and human services agencies, had an average of forty employees and five operating sites. All offered health insurance. Not surprisingly, nutrition fared better than physical activity in organizational support. Of fifteen physical-activity-promoting organizational practices assessed at baseline, only two were embraced by a majority of sites: support for casual dress at work and for standing and fidgeting at meetings. Half were endorsed by either none of the agencies or by just one agency. But three of fifteen practices encouraging healthy eating were in place in two-thirds or more of the agencies—functional water fountains, functional water coolers, and nutrient-rich food at every meeting—and five more were supported by at least a quarter of agencies. However, the most common response to questions about *formal* company policies supporting physical activity or healthy eating was zero percent, meaning that only a handful of sites had institutionalized these wellness practices. This ranged from zero percent (allowing activity during paid company time or accommodating activity with flexible hours) to 62 percent (offering nutrition classes). Workplaces with more physical-activity-supportive policies tended to have more healthy-eating-supportive policies.

Organizational wellness practices and policies were linked to worker health. Allowing physical activity on paid company time and several other practices were associated with employee physical activity levels, as was one form of social support—when people reported that their co-workers suggested or demonstrated an activity such as a new dance step, they were likely to be more active. Allowing paid time for exercise was also marginally associated with smaller waists. Offering healthy foods in vending machines or at meetings was associated with smaller waists and lower weights.

Because of inconsistent data-collection procedures (that's the purpose of a pilot test—to work out the kinks), we only consider the measurements from the last group of sites really reliable. Among these eight sites (six intervention sites implementing the changes, and two control sites for comparison purposes) with 130 workers, we demonstrated that the intervention produced small decreases in blood pressure and stabilized weight. In other words, the workers at the sites implementing the changes dropped their blood pressure slightly (–1.3) and didn't gain weight, while the blood pressure of those not implementing the changes increased a little (+1.2) and they gained weight (+0.4 BMI units, or three to four pounds). These findings are preliminary—we're still analyzing the data.

In 2008, we received a subsequent grant from the same federal agency to ramp up to a full-scale study in sixty to eighty sites involving about 1,500 people. We're delivering the intervention to the second group of seven sites at the time of this writing.

Adaptation of Lift Off! *to Youth Populations*
Rebranded as Instant Recess

So far this chapter, I've been talking about getting adults to build exercise into their lives with the organizational efforts and encouragement of their leaders and peers. For kids, I support getting college and pro athletes involved. The athletes don't need to come to the classroom or playground. Kids, of course, react well even when their heroes are on the small screen, with supporting materials.

In running any sort of program like this for schools, you have to take care to make it lean and mean: it has to be cost-efficient—classrooms are already strained for books and desks—and it needs to be minimally disruptive to already stretched budgets and constrained and overscheduled curricula.

I elected to team up with professional athletes, in part because UCLA studies have demonstrated that athletes are the second-largest category of role models among adolescents, behind family members (Yancey, Siegel, and McDaniel 2002). Having an athlete as a role model is comparable to having other types of "figure" role models (those not personally known to the teen) in its positive correlation with self-esteem, ethnic identity, and grades. Among white males in single-parent homes, choosing a sports figure correlated with decreased drug use. Plus, on the more obvious side, kids who emulate athletes tend to have higher physical activity levels. Our analyses of California Health Interview Survey data show an association between teens identifying an athlete as a role model and their engaging in a spectrum of protective behaviors, including exercising regularly, eating five or more daily servings of fruits and vegetables, not smoking or drinking alcohol, and not fighting at school (Yancey et al. 2010).

The *Lift Off!* model was adopted in 2006 by the newly formed non-profit Professional Athletes Council (PAC). PAC was founded by Allen Rossum, then of the NFL Atlanta Falcons, and Jerry Stackhouse, then of the NBA Dallas Mavericks, and managed by Shawn Wilson of SWI Consulting, who runs the philanthropic foundations of many of the athletes. Several of these foundations targeted obesity, kids' fitness, and diabetes, but were strictly locally focused. These athletes joined together to leverage their celebrity to draw national media attention, create a sensation (word of mouth, or buzz), and drive social norm change to fight childhood obesity. I was introduced to them by the executive director of the national Action for Healthy Kids non-profit and quickly became their chief scientific adviser or coach.

Prompted, in part, by our decision to reject an offer of $2 million from a beverage company, a sponsor of PAC's New York launch, Shawn and I worked over the first six months to develop a set of Principles of Engagement for Long-Term Success. This was an effort to stimulate a dialogue to assist the very different worlds of public health and sports to operate in a mutually respectful fashion, but in keeping with their respective and often diametrically opposed missions. Some of these principles follow:

1. To avoid conflicting missions, corporate sponsorship (displaying partnership names or logos) should ideally be restricted to health clubs, managed care organizations, groceries, sporting goods manufacturers and distributors, retail stores, and others whose profits will grow with the success of the project. Banks, law firms, and

other "cost neutral" enterprises are also eligible for sponsorship. Only logos for health-promoting product lines of other companies (such as food) should be permitted to be used in connection with the initiative.

2. Athletes should take a consistently positive stance in favor of health-promoting activities and avoid taking a negative stance (against highly profitable beer sales, for example, which are part of spectator sports' business model). A positive stance will also help them avoid charges of hypocrisy when players or franchises involved in the partnership also endorse fitness-compromising options such as cars, soda, or sedentary video games.

3. Projects should be essentially self-sustaining or turnkey: that is, they should build on the existing infrastructure (stadium space, product sales, IT capacity, Web site, PR, etc.), with most necessary management outsourced to public or nonprofit health or community service partners.

4. To best leverage their celebrity and visibility, athletes and sports franchises should consciously and conscientiously model healthy-eating and active-living policies and practices; they should take the lead by requesting a similar show of leadership by colleagues, partners, teammates, vendors, subcontractors, sponsors, grantees, community benefit recipients, and philanthropic beneficiaries such as youth programs.

PAC, the California Department of Public Health, and UCLA produced a prototype CD and DVD, the *Rossum Kick-Off Lift Off!* I adapted *Instant Recess* to target sports events and K–12 schools, with the aim of making prolonged sitting as socially unacceptable as drinking and driving, or smoking. We trademarked the concept after a presentation to executives of one of the national professional sports leagues because we feared it might be appropriated and co-opted for public relations with no real substance. The Los Angeles County Department of Public Health and the University of Pennsylvania–based African American Collaborative Obesity Research Network participated in vetting and testing various aspects of the *Instant Recess* adaptation, and plans for its implementation and evaluation. We also tested the *Instant Recess* concept and the first CD-DVD with children attending Paul Pierce and Baron Davis's Los Angeles Stars event at USC in August 2007 to document the kids' interest, willingness to participate, and accelerometer-measured levels of moderate to vigorous physical activity.

Allen Rossum is really running with the ball, as he did so well on the field, championing *Instant Recess* with schools and youth programs as a part of his philanthropy's Game Time Tour, mostly by reaching out to kids and training them to implement activity breaks. However, he's also championed the cause on the public health lecture circuit, attending public health meetings, and creating stampedes of otherwise distinguished professionals clamoring for autographs on his *InstantRecess* CDs and DVDs. We shot some of the footage for that first *Instant Recess* DVD at the California Childhood Obesity meeting in Anaheim in January 2007, and watched attendees ignore the keynote address by former California state health officer and environmental health advocate Dr. Dick Jackson to line up in the back of the auditorium to get Allen's signature. And few of these folks even knew who Allen was! That was when he was with the Atlanta Falcons, well before his stint in California as a San Francisco 49er.

The organization's maturational process has presented ever-greater opportunities and challenges. The Principles of Engagement we'd set out may seem pretty straightforward but, in practice, it's a whole 'nother ballgame. That offer of $2 million early in PAC's evolution—turned down because of the beverage company's unwillingness to agree to exclude their main product logo in PAC marketing and promotion—was put back on the table. And since the athletes had yet to receive substantial matching funds from public health agencies or foundations to build PAC's infrastructure, this created a dilemma. They considered how much good they could do with that investment, compared with any tarnishing of the brand or undermining of their message because they were seen as being in bed with a soda manufacturer. Certainly having the organization fold would do nothing to arrest childhood obesity, and their survival as an organization could contribute a lot to the cause, but were increases in obesity likely to result from the company's co-branding of their activities? Of course as a public health professional, I weighed in on not taking the money, but mine was only one voice. And the reality is that, despite claims to the contrary, no one knows the answer to that question. So far, PAC's holding the line and refusing the bucks.

INSTANT RECESS LEAVES THE NEST

The more formal dissemination and evaluation of *Instant Recess* to schools and sports organizations began with early adopters captivated by Rossum's charm (and perhaps my data) at presentations or lectures. The early progression was from individual initiatives at isolated schools in Los Angeles, Phoenix, and Memphis to a pro franchise, the San Diego Padres, and a school district, Winston-Salem/Forsyth County Schools in North Carolina.

Champion School: Testing the Feasibility of Instant Recess *in Resource-Challenged Schools*

Instant Recess was pilot-tested during the 2007–08 school year at a charter in Phoenix, Arizona, serving a low-income, ethnic minority student population. In order to better evaluate its influence, the school introduced *Instant Recess* first to half of the grade levels—K, 2, 4, and 6—at the beginning of the fall semester, and then to the rest at the beginning of the spring semester. They hosted a "Think You Got Moves?" contest, submitted a DVD of the three finalists' entries, and performed their moves with Rossum and other pro athletes attending the 2008 Super Bowl. Principal Carolyn Sawyer commented that "our students and teachers love [*Instant Recess*] and are getting quite good at it." Coach Clinton (Junior) Taylor, former UCLA football standout who runs the school's PE program, observed that kids exposed to *Instant Recess* learned exercise routines faster, and performed better on skills and endurance tests such as wall climbing. Many teachers told us they loved it:

- "It's a good use of time because it gets kids excited, gives them a boost of energy, wakes them up . . . "
- "Girls, especially, perform better in physical education because *Instant Recess* exercises build their confidence."
- "Kids are taking ownership—bringing their own music and trying out moves."
- "I really enjoy doing the exercise with the students. I feel more energized."

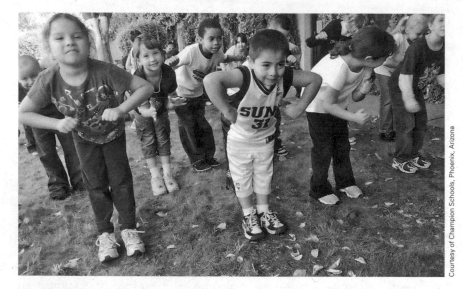

Courtesy of Champion Schools, Phoenix, Arizona

Figure 19.   Champion School students flex their muscles in combining *Instant Recess* with a strong PE curriculum.

- *"Instant Recess* is a great activity for the students. They get excited and can't wait to do it each day. It even helps students work together as a team and help each other out."
- "Students never let us forget to implement *Instant Recess.*"
- "They correct each other if they are not doing it right and teach *Instant Recess* to new students."
- "Kids are taking ownership—they want to dance to it, do it double time and infuse *Instant Recess* with their own moves."

Students said:

- "I think the *Instant Recess* is good for stretching out and exercising the kids to keep our muscles strong. I think it would be good to have all the kids around the world do it."
- "I like the modified jumping jacks because we don't have to pick up our feet!"
- "Makes me feel strong!"
- "I think it's cool!"

- "I love the *Instant Recess* because it gave me energy throughout the day."
- "When we did the *Instant Recess* I thought it was good because we got to work out but we did not get that sweaty."
- "Enjoyable. The part I like most was all of the moving around."
- "I thought it was a lot of fun. It was way better than sitting down in class all of the time."
- "The DVD was fun because you kept marching the whole time, but I wish we could learn new moves after a while."
- "I liked the music because it was easy to move to."
- "The music was good and made me feel fun and silly when I was doing the exercises."
- "I think that it would be awesome if we kept it going, and I think that none of them were too hard."
- "I thought it was fun and the best. I think other schools should do it so they can become more active."
- "I think that overall it's a good workout."
- "Yes, it will keep us healthy and active."
- "Yes, because it is fun to do in class rather than outside."

Winston-Salem/Forsyth County Schools: Bringing Instant Recess *to Scale at the District Level*

We've taken the next step as a follow-on to this individual school pilot test by scaling up to the school district level in the Winston-Salem/ Forsyth County Schools (WSFCS). The introduction of *Instant Recess* was timely because of a two-year-old regulatory policy of the North Carolina Department of Education mandating a minimum of 30 minutes of moderate to vigorous physical activity daily for all K–8 students. WSFCS goes even further, strongly encouraging schools to provide up to 225 activity minutes per week. WSFCS schools were struggling to meet the mandated requirements until they were introduced to *Instant Recess* at a School Health Advisory Council meeting. The school superintendent quickly bought into the idea. I collaborated with Melicia Whitt-Glover and the WSFCS in securing Robert Wood Johnson Foundation funding for an initial evaluation of whether *Instant Recess* helped schools adhere to the health policy and whether kids would do it. Participants included students in seven elementary schools and eight after-school programs. Pre- and post-implementation data showed significant improvements in participation in moderate to vigorous physical activity among students and a significant increase in on-task behavior (the percentage of students who were paying attention in class), compared to controls. At the time of this writing, the WSFCS system was seeking ways to roll *Instant Recess* out to middle schools.

A secondary and complementary aim was to make exercise breaks an integral part of high school, community college, and university sporting events to embed the intervention in the local culture and increase its diffusion and dissemination. Our UCLA CDC disparities center provided a seed grant for this purpose to augment the school day–focused funding. However, because of a cascade of administrative changes and bureaucratic snafus, the CDC funds have yet to be released and full implementation of this component has been delayed. In concert with our earlier collaboration targeting black churches to incorporate *Instant Recess* breaks, the eventual goal is to include *Instant Recess* in enough venues so that Winston-Salem metro area residents (population, about three hundred thousand) have an opportunity to participate in at least one activity break every day.

Duarte, California: Institutionalizing Instant Recess as a Symbol of City Commitment to Wellness

Over the past ten years, I've trained a number of public employees in California in conducting *Lift Off!*s at conferences and meetings for various local and state government programs and initiatives such as Women, Infants, and Children (WIC), Head Start, and the Nutrition Network that funded the first *Lift Off!* CD and DVD. The Duarte parks and rec director, Donna Georgino, attended one of these sessions. Championed by city councilmember Lois Gaston-Greene and Donna, Duarte (a city of about twenty-five thousand near Pasadena) installed recess breaks in its twice monthly city council meetings in 2003, and have been going strong ever since. And they didn't put them at the end of the evening when only the diehards are still there. The 3-minute "fitness warm-ups" are front and center on the meeting agenda, right after the flag salute and moment of reflection. Donna is always the backup leader, but they may also get the police chief, city manager, or someone from the audience to select the type of activity.

Lois likens the breaks to "seatbelts, so the younger generation can pick up healthy habits early." She hails from Taylor, Arkansas, a tiny town on the train route from Hope, Arkansas, to Shreveport, Louisiana. Like most other women of her generation—the front end of the baby boom—Lois acknowledges that exercise is not her thing. However, she grew up walking to get from place to place and picking and savoring huckleberries and other fruits right off the trees. Walking has continued to be a regular part of her lifestyle.

And the recess breaks are just the tip of the iceberg. She's rightfully proud of the fact that under her decade-long leadership, physical activity has become embedded in every health program as a central prevention strategy. For example, the dietitians don't just lecture people about healthy eating—they take parents on walking tours of the grocery store to help them identify nutrient-rich selections that fit their budget. The after-school programs include active recreation along with healthy meals and refreshments. Summer camps feature physically active games, nutrient-rich meals and treats, and kid-friendly MyPyramid nutrition education lessons. Midnight basketball is central to the city's violence prevention approach.

And Lois has worked across regions and sectors, teaming with school board member Reina Diaz, for instance, to make sure that the city's monolingual Spanish-speaking populations don't get left behind when it comes to prevention. For example, at school fund-raisers, vendors are selling fresh fruit cups or watermelon rather than churros. As head of the California Contract Cities Association, an organization of elected officials in the state, she's beginning to see the spread of the message of health consciousness and prevention—and action on the policy and practice front as a result. Lois was nearing the end of her term on the council at the time of this writing, but her legacy will undoubtedly endure.

Orange County Health Care Agency: Instant Recess—
an Inexpensive Employee Benefit and More!

Events surrounding the Orange County Health Care Agency's adoption
of *Lift Off!* led to the agency's emergence as a shining example of how
to do it right. The health promotion program supervisor there, Kelly
Broberg, heard about our *Lift Off!* training seminars from one of my
doctoral students—her employee Raúl Sobero. Kelly returned from the
training excited about the science supporting the approach. Her enthusiasm was contagious, spreading to her division manager, Amy Buch, and
several other health professionals in the agency's leadership, including
the agency's deputy director of public health services, who also had a
background in health education. I interviewed Kelly and Amy for this
book, and I can tell you that their passion's still palpable. Having years
of experience in trying—mostly unsuccessfully like the rest of us—to
educate and counsel people to be active, they embraced the concept
that the real benefit to the agency would come from participation by
otherwise sedentary employees unlikely to devote their free time to such
a pursuit. They were well aware that incentives like subsidized gym
memberships generally don't work, especially for sedentary folks. So
in pitching the intervention, they stressed the importance of providing
paid time to do it.

Shortly after Kelly attended the training in the spring of 2007, Eric
Handler became the new agency health officer when longtime health
officer Mark Horton left to become the head of California's state public
health department. Eric requested suggestions from his management
team for practical and inexpensive evidence-based employee wellness
interventions. Kelly and Amy floated *Lift Off!* among a number of
other ideas, and, along with CDC-style stairwell renovations, it stuck.
Other selling points were OCHCA's desire, as Orange County's largest
employer, to model the organizational behavior for other companies, and
the program's minimal cost to the employer. Even if managers weren't
convinced of the benefits to the bottom line, the program represented a
goodwill gesture to improve employee morale in tough economic times.

Around this same time, the whole agency was going through safety training. Kelly, tapping into her background in injury prevention, was able to hitch *Lift Off!* to this effort in a key meeting with human relations managers. This reframing was important, because initial management concerns centered on the possibility of increased injuries associated with the exercises. (In the three years since project inception, no injuries attributable to the activity breaks have been reported.)

The preparation process has been extensive and wide-ranging, bottom up as well as top down. For example, timing and location of the breaks were carefully selected to minimize disruption and head off disgruntlement of nonparticipating employees. Managers anticipated that some would argue that they should be able to use the 10 paid minutes for other purposes, but division heads stuck to their guns on the science—that this was the wellness strategy that had been demonstrated to benefit both the individual and the organization.

In May 2008, after a full year of securing support throughout the organization's leadership, then preparation and piloting, the department issued a formal policy permitting daily 10-minute *Lift Off!*s on paid county time. The agency has since arranged for *Lift Off!* training on site, with about fifty staff trained to date.

Support is provided for the newly trained: veteran Health Promotion Division staff members make themselves available to co-lead breaks with the new champions to build their confidence. Regularly scheduled activity breaks, announced by e-mail in advance, and a blast immediately beforehand, occur in four of the main buildings housing the health department staff, with participants representing many different departments and programs. Taking advantage of opportunities for visibility and broader exposure, the agency's Public Health Week celebration in 2009 featured the "largest *Lift Off!* ever in the OC," hosted in a quad between county buildings during a county board of supervisors hearing. The agency's Health Promotion unit set up a table with copies of its *Lift Off!* policy and frequently asked questions (FAQ) sheets to take advantage of the traffic from other county agencies, with sign-up sheets for those interested in being trained. Next up, an on-site train-the-trainer session for the health promotion staff, to accommodate the demand for training among OCHCA staff and speed dissemination. The OCHCA has a waiting list and wants to be able to train people immediately upon request.

San Diego Padres' FriarFit Initiative:
Developing a Pro Sports Model for Instant Recess

In 2008, the San Diego Padres became the first professional sports team to adopt *Instant Recess* and other organizational policy and practice changes in its routine operations after I was hired by a foundation to help the Padres develop a broad-based childhood obesity prevention initiative, FriarFit. My team at UCLA created and choreographed an *Instant Recess* break for the initiative, with nine baseball moves representing each of the nine innings in baseball. *Instant Recess* breaks were led by the club's Pad Squad—and by a celebrity or Padres player—during the pregame shows at ten of the thirteen family-focused Sunday games during the pilot year and, on occasion, at other youth events, like baseball clinics.

The Padres also produced and showed public service announcements featuring players, cheerleaders, and former players on the jumbo screens during games and on the team's cable network affiliate. In conjunction with the state health department's Project LEAN (Leaders Encouraging Activity and Nutrition), we provided training, resource materials, technical assistance and support, and incentives to thirty-nine teachers and administrators from economically challenged local school districts to conduct the in-class breaks and mobilize school wellness committees to advocate for physical activity promotion strategies. Those included recess before lunch and standards to require at least 50 percent of physical education time in moderate to vigorous activity. Ten nutrient-rich items were upgraded or added to the ballpark menu, including sweet-pepper hummus with baked pita chips, fresh fruit cups, yogurt parfaits, Asian salads, and grilled veggie dogs and burgers on whole grain buns. An informational Web page with its own link was created. Media coverage included several TV and radio networks, along with local newspapers. The team was given a leadership and community service award by the county board of supervisors to highlight national Physical Fitness and Sports Month.

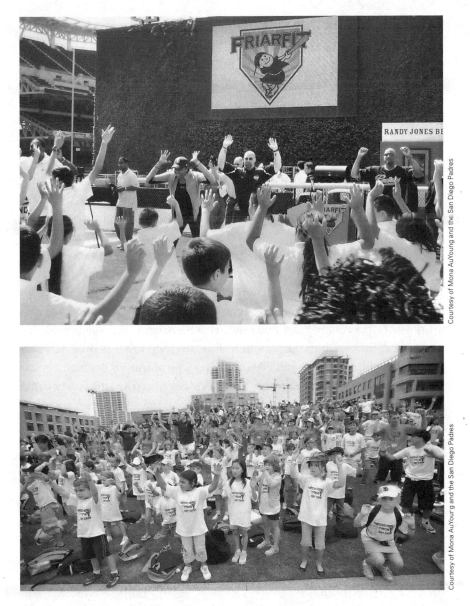

Figures 20 and 21. FriarFit Launch with the San Diego Padres.

During the second season, teacher training sessions were hosted at the ballpark and an interactive Web site was launched with plans for Web-based interscholastic competitions for such prizes as game tickets or visits by players or cheerleaders to lead *Instant Recess* breaks on site.

We learned many lessons during the first season, some the hard way. For one thing, we came to appreciate that favorable publicity and recognition accrues to all parties involved, but the likelihood of criticism should anything go wrong falls disproportionately on the team. This presents a greater risk to the franchise than is typical for community relations projects and a greater degree of uncertainty about the gain from success. It also became obvious that public health aims have to be addressed in ways that are financially viable and that deliver tangible value for a profit-making concern, in this case, enhanced or new product sales, ticket sales, public and community relations, and brand marketing, or "media impressions." The importance of opening a dialogue to clarify the terms of engagement became increasingly apparent. This was an ongoing process, not an outcome. The Principles of Engagement for Long-Term Success hammered out in building the PAC, as outlined earlier in this chapter, came in very handy as a jumping-off point. Carving out a middle or common ground was critical because athletes became involved in the initiative as a part of their obligation to the franchise's public relations and community outreach efforts. This created an even greater chance that their commercial marketing engagements would conflict with the initiative's mission and undermine its message.

We're now beginning to see passive diffusion of the Padres model. Major League Baseball's national office requested the FriarFit materials and documents as a part of the R&D of MLBFit. Some teams began implementing initiatives similar to FriarFit during the 2009 season. For example, the LA Dodgers have added some of the same healthy food items offered by the Padres and have included "follow along exercises" broadcast over the huge DodgerVision screen to engage children and willing adults.

We're also engaged in active dissemination through our CDC Center of Excellence in the Elimination of Disparities grant. The WNBA Los Angeles Sparks signed on to pilot the project during the 2009 season, developing *SPARKing* Motion in conjunction with our center and the

Los Angeles County Department of Public Health. Didn't hurt that Sparks' president, Kristin Bernert, knew Jeff Overton, the Padres' former executive vice president, who was instrumental in getting FriarFit off the ground. On August 30, 2009, the Sparks hosted the first in-game *Instant Recess* break during their half-time show with political and public health leaders working out on the floor with their two cheerleader groups, the SparKids and Ole Skool Crew, also featured in the DVD. The *SPARKing* Motion *Instant Recess* break consisted of basketball moves we created for ten of the players on the active roster, including Tina "the Thompson Tip-Off" and Candace "Power Jam" Parker. DeLisha Milton-Jones, a real sweetheart to work with and a philanthropist in her own right, did the voiceover for the thousand audio CDs we distributed that night to the crowd at the Staples Center.

California's Women, Infants, and Children Program's FitWIC & WIC Walks the Talk

In the case of California's Women, Infants, and Children (WIC), a nutrition program for low-income pregnant women and their children, administrative changes have favorably influenced wellness initiative institutionalization.

WIC clinics in California began implementing a wellness initiative, FitWIC, a decade ago. Recess breaks were a prominent part of this initiative, which began with a randomized, controlled pilot study in three sites—one intervention clinic each in Southern California, Oakland, and Sacramento.

We found that compared with control sites, the initiative significantly

- increased perceived workplace support for staff physical activity (96 versus 58 percent) and healthy food choices (85 versus 28 percent);

- changed the types of foods served during meetings (72 percent versus 24 percent) and the priority placed on physical activity in the workplace (96 versus 71 percent);

- increased the amount of encouragement that parents and families got to be physically active (64 percent versus 35 percent) and raised the sensitivity of staff in handling weight-related issues (92 versus 58 percent).

In focus groups, staff members indicated that they felt they had something to offer parents to help get their children active, instead of just telling them their kids were fat.

These positive pilot outcomes, published as an article called "Walking the Talk" (Crawford et al. 2004) in a special themed issue of the *American Journal of Public Health,* led to the rollout of a statewide wellness initiative, WIC Walks the Talk. The California WIC Association has 3,500 workers in more than 650 sites serving 1.4 million families each month. A recent wellness survey of 1,500 WIC staff about their wellness awareness, concerns, and involvement found that more than 75 percent responded that it was very likely or somewhat likely that they'd use a 5-minute break for activity if it were offered. The activity breaks fit under one of ten steps to assist WIC agencies in becoming certified as Well WIC Worksites—not bad, number two on the list behind promoting and ensuring the accessibility of healthy food options (after all, it is a nutrition program). However, as the saying goes, the spirit is willing, but the flesh is weak! I'm encouraged that many of the agencies are recognizing the need to institutionalize activity breaks as an anchor to get everyone to do a little something, along with spurring people to do more. The level of investment in promoting recess model strategies will ultimately determine the overall success of the project. This has proved to be true at L. L. Bean over twenty-plus years of nurturing a culture of wellness.

Fortunately, businesspeople and entrepreneurs don't require the same level of evidence for decision making as academic researchers. This can be helpful in persuading them to try something promising, especially if their competitors seem to be having some success. Same thing for elected or appointed public officials—what the mayor in the next town or the senator in their fraternity is doing is much more compelling for them than stats. A compelling story is worth a thousand numbers. However, companies or locales are rarely willing to spend the time, money, or other resources necessary to rigorously evaluate wellness initiatives. Mainly for this reason, documentation of a positive effect on the bottom line is rarely possible and even seemingly effective efforts are often eliminated when there's a fiscal downturn. That's truly an understatement for the situation in 2010.

WHERE WE'RE GOING FROM HERE

The political traction in environmental solutions to the obesity and chronic-disease epidemic is in childhood obesity prevention and control. However, intervening only with children will not solve the problem. It's late in the game, and a lot of damage has already been done, so small-scale fixes won't to get us to the tipping point where large-scale social change becomes inevitable. Social norms have to change in order for the adults who govern children's lives—and all of our lives—to make the decisions and model the behaviors that drive meaningful, substantive, and widespread organizational practice and policy change, and regulatory and legislative policy change. The motto of Tom Friedman, the *New York Times* columnist and author of *Hot, Flat, and Crowded,* is "Change your leaders, not your light bulbs. Because what leaders do is rewrite the rules" (2008). Yet we so often perseverate in letting our leaders (us!) off the hook by emphasizing personal responsibility. We need to override this compulsion of ours arising from our rugged individualist, libertarian value system that puts the onus on individuals to make changes themselves, one by one. Lori Dorfman, who heads the Berkeley Media Studies Center, has been making this point for years in pushing to reframe the public obesity dialogue with messages targeting decision makers rather than consumers or end users.

The only environmental solutions that are currently politically tenable are budget-neutral or demonstrably cost-effective ones. The recess model is such a solution that provides a starting point within the decision-making latitude of a host of early adopter leaders—leaders who might be persuaded to look in the mirror and realize that small but effective changes are within their grasp. And that these changes can further their own organizational aims. Joe Donnelly, head of the PAAC study at University of Kansas profiled earlier in this chapter, ended up exceeding his recruitment goals by 50 percent. "When our sales marketing pitch to schools shifted from health [improvement] to classroom management and academic achievement, we got their attention."

It's also time for the spark plugs to go to work—those of us committed to population-wide physical activity promotion who have the passion and expertise to market recess to these leaders—to sell them on the idea that these wellness practices and policies are in their organizational best interest, and may even offer a competitive advantage. Such widespread small changes could produce sufficient momentum to begin reintegrating physical activity into daily life. As a society, we really must take on some of the responsibility or cost for achieving and maintaining health and fitness—to shift a part of the burden from the individual to the systemic level. The cost of not doing so has become prohibitive, both individually and collectively.

The recess model of reintegrating brief bouts of activity into everyday routine, with its ease of cultural targeting and adaptation and of audiovisual electronic media delivery, is the aerobics of the twenty-first century. Recess is an updated exercise prescription for an increasingly overscheduled, ethnically diverse, multicultural, media- and information-technology-driven global postmodern society. Its emergence in settings dominated by female and ethnic minority population segments at high risk for sedentariness, helps make the case for this approach as an important step toward arresting and reversing our epidemic of physical inactivity.

SEVEN A Glimpse into the Future: How the Recess Model Sparked a Physical Activity Movement

So far, I've laid out the challenges and opportunities presented by the twin epidemics of obesity and sedentariness. Some of it's been pretty depressing stuff. So as a reward for sticking it out, join me on a visit to the future I envision that doesn't have to be sci-fi.

America made a giant leap toward promoting a fit and healthy populace at the end of the first decade of the twenty-first century. It was ripe for radical transformation, and it signaled that desire in the election of Barack Obama. The multinational economic crisis was threatening to rupture our health care system. Growing instability in the Middle East was escalating our discomfort with our heavy dependence on foreign oil. Rapid acceleration of global warming in plain sight combined with a man-made deepwater drilling catastrophe in astounding proportions were erasing the complacency of even the most cynical Americans about resource conservation and environmental preservation.

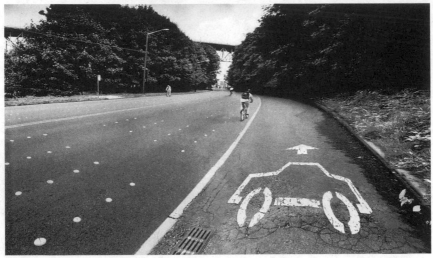

© Bob Peterson/Seattle

Figure 22.   Redesigned highways envision a very different, very active future.

There was little choice except to adopt health reform, and not merely health *care* reform. The second decade of the twenty-first century witnessed the development of the political will to create an activity-friendly infrastructure, sparked by widespread adoption of *Instant Recess* practices and policies. The built environment is now being reshaped by the steady erosion of complacency. As population fitness levels improve and physical activity opportunities become more valued, social controls like aggressive regulation and legislation have tilted toward mass transit over private transportation. The result is a dramatically changed landscape that was once only dreamed of by hard-core green activists, community redevelopment experts, healthy-cities advocates, and hiking and biking enthusiasts. And a vibrant, productive, energized and reinvigorated America.

WHY *INSTANT RECESS* WORKED

As we moved into the 2010s, the societal toll of rampant sedentariness was finally fully recognized, and physical activity promotion came to be appreciated as the linchpin of obesity control policy. Skyrocketing health care costs, due in large part to the inactivity-related epidemics of diabetes, Alzheimer's, and obesity, were also major drivers of society's newfound willingness to redirect resources to prevention. It had become clear, even to the legions of late-adopter leaders, that aging baby boomers and unfit Gen Xers would continue to drive the medical care system to the breaking point if major change was not undertaken. The Gen Xers in their late thirties and forties, who should have been heading for peak productivity in the prime of their lives, were actually becoming ill and disabled in alarming numbers. This created a leadership vacuum that was partially filled by the healthiest boomers postponing their retirement, along with US-educated first-generation immigrants from the developing world. The health of the Gen Yers was also doolining rapidly and already substantially worse than that of the previous several generations. This brought to the forefront doomsday scenarios of the toppling of America as the leader of the free world, a position it had just reclaimed during the first Obama administration.

As is often the case, different triggers activated different population segments. Climbing rates of Alzheimer's disease undoubtedly precipitated dramatic attitudinal shifts among the affluent, who'd enjoyed excellent health and unparalleled longevity for generations. With no substantial drug treatment on the horizon, physical activity was one of the few known preventive measures. Fear of Alzheimer's, in fact, marked the tipping point at which decision-maker self-interest factored into this cascade of events, much as the high rates of breast and prostate cancer in their ranks directed dollars toward cancer control in the 1990s. The obesity of the majority of children, even in middle-income communities, was inescapable and embarrassing to the American elite. The "stealth intervention" of soaring gas prices did the trick among the regular Janes and Joes. Swelling trains and buses to the bursting point, their outcry for investment in mass transit was deafening, and politicians sped projects that had languished for years from "shovel ready" to completion at a breakneck pace. In the nation's crumbling and foreclosure-blighted inner cities, the ravages of diabetes caused people to take to the streets in droves. This disease had emerged as the number one killer of adolescents and younger adults—surpassing HIV/AIDS and homicide, and diabetes-related amputations had replaced gunshot wounds as the main reason young men ended up in wheelchairs.

HOW *INSTANT RECESS* WORKED

Much as the rapid spread of policies and practices banning smoking sparked the adoption of regulatory tobacco control policies (such as requiring smoke-free workplaces to receive federal funding), *Instant Recess* permitted just about anyone to answer the call, representing an opportunity for immediate action that could engage the alarmed masses. *Instant Recess* sparked policy changes to promote physical activity, starting as mere incrementalist tweaking to provide modest incentives. But then momentum surged, producing aggressive legislation and regulations with strong incentives and disincentives, as well as monitoring and accountability provisions. These rebuilt the landscape of cities and suburbs.

Instant Recess and recess-type organizational practice and policy changes were appropriately framed and marketed to convince leaders across key sectors that the adoption of these changes served their organizational best interests. Practice-oriented research—increasingly the focus of federal public health funding agencies across the board—produced findings that fueled an avalanche of media attention. Media interest was also fueled by the involvement of outlets in that sector as employers and as purveyors of *Instant Recess* products and services.

The surge in *Instant Recess*'s diffusion in the 2010s catalyzed the emergence of physical activity as a cornerstone of obesity and chronic disease control. This surge was predicted by my theoretical model—the Meta-Volition Model (Yancey 2009).

In Theory

Thus far, I've described how to implement *Instant Recess*, what others are doing, and what outcomes they're finding, but not why it works. Now I'm going to delve into the "black box" of what's going on at the micro-level—inside the people and implementing organizations—and how that results in dissemination. Basically, I'm explaining in more detail why and how recess physical activity push policies and practices work.

The Meta-Volition Model, represented in figure 23, lays out the interaction of influences at different levels at which behavioral change can

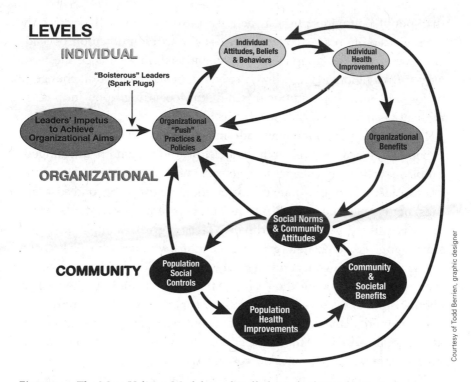

LEVELS

INDIVIDUAL

Figure 23. The Meta-Volition Model graphically lays out the interaction of influences at different levels at which behavior change can occur.

occur, from the individual and her or his social network to the organizational and then to the societal (economic, legal, and political systems). There's also an institutional level that I do not explicitly address (in sectors like education and religion, for example), but the model may be applied there as well. At each level of the model, participation builds and swells until it spills over to the next. Implicit in the model is that each level also feeds back into the previous ones, further swelling the spillover. For example, individual health improvements continue to spur the adoption of push practices by individuals more closely connected within a particular segment of an organization, say a work unit or committee, and by other segments across the organization, as word travels (see a detailed description of phases of change below). The model predicts that population-wide physical activity participation will occur only when society embraces collective efficacy and the motivation of leaders rewarded for accomplishing organizational aims—hence the term *meta-volition* (ibid.) as the primary driver of health behavioral change, a major shift from the traditional paradigm depending upon individual motivation and self-efficacy for this impetus.

Meta-volition explains how individual, organizational, and societal benefits may accrue even if individual attitudes remain unchanged. Employees choosing cheaper remote parking is one example. They may not consider it exercise, value the experience or benefits beyond cost savings, nor change their identity to reflect their more active status. Mark Fenton, walking guru extraordinaire, gives a great example: a stocky Harrisburg, Pennsylvania, government office worker who picked the dollar-a-day parking lot across a bridge from the downtown area, rather than paying $8 daily for the lot in his building (2009). But when asked about his newly acquired nonsedentary status, he was unaware that he was any more active, nor did he care about being active. It was strictly an economic decision—the $150 per month savings more than made up for the extra twenty minutes of required walking.

Here's a straightforward and concrete analogy—lifting a heavy weight. Your brain signals your intention to move the weight through a nerve, activating individual muscle fibers. After enough muscle fibers are recruited to help out, the muscle begins to contract. But one muscle's not usually enough to lift something heavy. So you have to recruit a sufficient number of muscles to contract in order to generate enough power to lift the weight. Granted this all occurs in microseconds, and the model's "fountain of change" takes a bit longer to flow.

The model's built on several established public health theories, including social cognitive theory, the diffusion of innovations, and social marketing. Social marketing, to which I devoted chapter 4, provides an overarching framework for voluntary behavioral change focused on exchange theory (Andreasen 1995). People want to be healthier, thinner, and fitter. But the cost is just more than most are willing to pay, and the rewards are too far in the future. The model offers a mechanism by which the costs may be lowered—you don't have to go out of your way, rock the boat, swim upstream . . . the behavioral change happens right where you already are doing something you consider worthwhile.

This default option concept is also central to behavioral economics, but that field developed in parallel with my change model and has been applied primarily to nutrition (for example, an individual is more likely to choose water over soda if the water is at eye level in the vending machine and the soda is at the bottom). Some rewards are immediate—camaraderie and social interaction with friends or co-workers, energy, stress relief, muscle relaxation, improved affect, and concentration. And because it occurs regularly, longer-term rewards begin to manifest—mood elevation, less exertion when doing ordinary things like climbing a flight of stairs, tightening the belt a notch.

The elements of social cognitive theory most pertinent to the Meta-Volition Model are incremental change and role modeling. The former means that people tend not to make changes in leaps and bounds but, rather, in small steps. The latter refers to learning from observing those we admire and aspire to be like, and emulating them—gaining some hands-on skills from the experience of participating. Both incremental learning and role modeling enhance confidence that we can accomplish what we set out to (Bandura 1989, 2004). For example, our UCLA studies identified athletes as the second-largest category of role models among adolescents, behind family members, and that ethnic minority youth choose ethnic minority role models (Yancey, Siegel, and McDaniel 2002; Yancey et al. 2010). Since emulating athletes is associated with higher physical activity levels, integrating brief bouts of *athlete-led* exercise into the classroom setting (even via DVDs and CDs) stands a good chance of getting children moving and improving their fitness levels. And athletes can help get everyone moving, since 70 percent of us follow at least one sport.

Another theory at the heart of the model is the "diffusion of innovations" (Rogers 2003). It addresses how leaders interested in effecting change can try out changes on a small scale first; how they can directly observe how well the changes are received and whether they fit into their organizational culture; and how they can weigh the relative advantage of a particular change over current practice. Diffusion of innovations posits that changes with characteristics like trialability are most likely to be adopted.

The Meta-Volition Model specifies six levels or phases of change: initiating, catalyzing, viral marketing, accelerating, anchoring, and institutionalizing. These phases are set in motion in different ways. Levels reflect progressively greater numbers of individuals and organizations or organizational units implementing the changes, eventually achieving a critical mass, or tipping point, from one level to the next.

The *initiating phase* of the model is *from leader to leader.* "Boisterous leaders," or spark plugs—charismatic, passionate leaders committed to population-wide physical activity promotion—market recess breaks to leaders of organizations in various sectors. Organizational leaders must respect these spark plugs as experts and colleagues—health professionals or researchers capable of helping them achieve their goals and offering a better way to get there. These spark plugs are the human catalysts of the changes that follow, as recess breaks are the behavioral catalysts.

The *catalyzing phase* to get the ball rolling is *from the organization to the individual.* Push practices like dance breaks and walking meetings operate kind of under the radar, framed as an energy booster or stress reliever—paid time to stretch and loosen up, rather than some obligation imposed from on high—to get people moving regularly without their really equating it with exercise. Because the changes are the default option, most people participate. Of course, active participation is voluntary, but sitting out, the other option, is inconvenient, goes against the flow, makes the person stand out as not being part of the group. Most people find thinking and weighing alternative actions draining. They either don't possess the cognitive processing power or summoning it up takes energy they elect to spend on higher-priority issues, not those they consider trivial. After all, energy's a finite quantity and a precious resource, and it tends to be rationed, from a behavioral economist's perspective (Thaler and Sunstein 2008). At least past the age of thirty! A person's own physiology, along with the social aspects, reinforce the activity—they have some fun, wake up a little, and get a bit of an energy boost. Next thing they know, in a couple weeks' time, they feel less taxed when going about their everyday activities and less intimidated by a little exertion—they take the stairs to get to the meeting rather than waiting for the elevator to go up a flight or two, and don't grumble as much about playing catch in the yard with their kids or taking the dog for a walk at the end of a long day.

Then the *viral marketing phase—from individual to organization*—kicks in. People start a buzz about the new break, spreading the word through their social circles both at work and outside work. This primes the pump. When people hear about recess breaks going on in other areas or departments discussed in glowing terms, they're unconsciously primed or disposed to view a subsequent opportunity to participate favorably. People in nearby divisions or work units encounter them doing their recess activities and, after a round or two of teasing, start noticing those folks have a little pep in their step at the end of the day. Sooner or later, recess participants drop a size or pull their belts in a notch. This not only gives them a sense of accomplishment but also gets noticed by their co-workers, friends, and families, kicking up the word of mouth beyond their immediate circles. As people start to feel a little better, they talk to others, and others notice the change. Maybe they even get an unexpected compliment on a routine visit to their doc when their blood pressure's down a bit and their good (HDL) cholesterol's up some. A little low-key bragging creates more buzz in their immediate circle of co-workers, friends, and family. Positive strokes are very reinforcing now from multiple segments of the social network.

Of course, bosses aren't immune to informal communication through their own social networks. They're starting to see some improvements in attitude: Less complaining and gossiping and more getting done. People who typically call in sick every other Monday showing up like they're supposed to. More work assignments turned in on time. Helping out without being asked. And bosses socialize with bosses in other depart-ments at work and outside the workplace. This heralds the start of the *accelerating phase: from organization to organization*. Anything that seems to be giving someone a leg up is bound to attract attention and, next thing you know, they're being hit up by others to find out what's going on and how to get it going where they work. Things are really rolling now. Communication of benefits to the organization is starting to pop up at conferences and meetings over lunch—pie charts and growth curves in their presentations inexplicably reflecting positive trends. Actually, not inexplicably. People are more alert, not checking out at the end of the day, not taking off just to use up their sick days. More work's getting done, and the higher-ups are now impressed and fully engaged.

Formal recognition begins to come in the form of monitoring and publishing productivity stats. Innovations attract media coverage, elevating the stature of the innovation and those associated with it, accelerating dissemination. Word spreads between sectors. The *anchoring phase* is *from the organization to the community.* Community attitudes and norms change. Public tolerance for sedentary behaviors erodes, like smoking, littering, not recycling, or drinking and driving. Political will builds and puts pressure on appointed and elected officials to act, leading to the development of population social controls (rules that direct and constrain behavior) and heralding the *institutionalizing phase, from the community to the individual.* New regulations are established, memorialized, and implemented, and new laws are enacted. The changes are now institutionalized or ingrained in the societal fabric. They are formally monitored and enforced, imposing serious consequences for violations, like confinement or the loss of certain privileges. Moreover, they are socially enforced and reinforced.

In Practice

Let's go back to our time machine—and forward to the year 2020: our optimistic look into newly fit 2010s America.

Not surprisingly, just as protecting kids from exposure to secondhand smoke is what turned the tide in anti-tobacco policy, so the will to stem the tide of childhood obesity brought about the shift in public policy to promote physical activity and avert sedentariness.

School

Instant Recess first gained traction in the public schools in economically challenged areas because it was cheap and easy and produced immediate results. The economic downturn of 2000–10 meant that a lot of areas were in that camp! Structured activity breaks represented a more feasible and sustainable practice in these schools, with their overcrowded classrooms, teachers pressed into instruction on topics outside their specialization, high teacher turnover, multiethnic and multicultural student populations, and lower levels of adherence to PE duration and quality mandates.

Activity breaks had begun to attract some attention in several states around 2008 because a few state and local school districts imposed minimum daily activity requirements for students. The North Carolina Department of Education's Healthy Active Children Policy, for example, required 30 minutes of physical activity over and above that occurring during phys ed classes. There were holdouts, however. Schools in low-income neighborhoods resisted the policies because of the need to identify, digest, and deliver written curricula outlining the activity breaks, and because the curricula didn't resonate culturally for their students.

But *Instant Recess* offered several advantages over doing nothing, or implementing the policies as recommended:

- Stressed and overburdened teachers got a brief breather.
- Teachers and other staff participated with the kids, bolstering their own energy levels and mood.
- *Instant Recess* came with a built-in cultural compatibility and adaptability.
- Delivery of the intervention by CD and DVD took the onus of preparing and executing the lessons off the classroom teachers, most of whom did not have any PE training or skills.
- Teachers and other staff who were sports fans or pop culture aficionados were excited by the involvement of pro athletes and teams, and therefore more enthusiastic about *Instant Recess*.
- The approach fit into different activities in any given school (from regular classrooms to interscholastic games to standardized testing periods), between schools and school districts, and beyond—to after-school programs, workplaces, churches, and sporting events.

Meantime, claims that *Instant Recess* competed with instructional time were easily debunked by overwhelming research showing that more physical activity improved test scores and grades. Even recalcitrant teachers and principals became fans when they saw that exercise made kids behave and perform better. (Ever notice how cranky your dogs get when a few days go by without a walk?)

Sports

The natural alliance of the sports and fitness industry and physical activity promotion embraced *Instant Recess*. Executives immediately and intuitively understood the dual, synergistic opportunities for advancing a philanthropic mission *and* selling tickets, logo merchandise, sports and fitness equipment, stadium advertising space, and corporate sponsorships. They'd figured out how to better leverage their existing assets—popular locations, easy media draws, electronic media production capabilities, abundant audio and video clips, cheerleader squads, school visits—along with their dollars. Compared with the typical donations to charitable causes, support for *Instant Recess* brought their franchises greater stature, visibility, and community team spirit and delivered a much greater health impact. They also recognized that better fitness levels among their future prospects, gifted youthful athletes, could help in the recruitment and development of new talent. Not to mention expanding the pipeline by attracting the best athletes to their sport and team.

At sporting events where activity breaks were incorporated into the pregame and halftime shows, including those at the high school and college levels, the media coverage and word of mouth set off a chain reaction spurring more recess breaks in various communities. The involvement of professional athletes and teams made the recess breaks hip and fashionable.

Philanthropy

Foundations, particularly those focused on health, have a mission to seed innovation. They tend to be more nimble and less risk averse than other health entities, leveraging smaller short-term investments with the expectation that successful demonstration projects will be adopted and institutionalized by like government or medical care institutions. The growth of physical gaming with the nurturance and support of foundations had been an indicator of the opportunity for spurring the diffusion of an approach or innovation. But there are some notable differences between promoting physical activity through physical video gaming and doing it with recess breaks.

Many health foundations were exposed to *Instant Recess* at conferences and regional collaboration meetings, and by the HEAL (Healthy Eating Active Living) Convergence, a special foundation network formed by several large foundations to address the obesity epidemic. Beginning in smaller cities and counties, these foundations pulled in willing partners like hospitals and local government agencies, and brought *Instant Recess* projects to local baseball farm teams, semipro hockey teams, community college sports teams, race tracks, county fairs, traveling carnivals, and other popular regular events. This helped recess breaks spread from large metropolitan areas to small and medium-sized communities throughout the US.

Government

State and local governments were poised and ready for *Instant Recess*. They were often the largest employers in a given locale, with significant ethnic and socioeconomic diversity. In 2010, Los Angeles County employed more than 120,000 people full time, and the city of Los Angeles employed 40,000. Three-quarters were people of color, and most were women. More than a third were over forty, two-thirds earned less than $50,000 per year, and half had been on the local payroll for more than fifteen years.

Not only did these factors make such government workforces ideal for *Instant Recess*, but the nature of the bureaucracy meant the benefits of these changes were regularly and meticulously monitored, documented, and scrutinized. Extended average lengths of service ensured not only adequate exposure time, but also time to reap the economic benefits of improved employee health status. Furthermore, among their staff were a disproportionate number of gatekeepers, opinion leaders, and decision makers at various levels from grassroots to elected and appointed leadership, particularly direct providers of human services. Personally benefiting from daily participation in recess breaks favorably influenced their decisions for and about their clients, workers, and citizenry from the standpoint of physical activity promotion. People became vocal and passionate in asserting that it was no longer acceptable to be cooped up for hours on end in meeting rooms, carrels, cubicles, offices, and other work spaces, no different from the bitching and moaning that would be precipitated by serving only meat and potatoes or permitting smoking.

Two things didn't change. Local TV stations still loved to roll when kids were involved. And politicians jumped on the bandwagon, rushing to put activity breaks in every public appearance, especially at schools and youth events, in their own field offices to sport their "walking the talk" at every turn, and on city council and school board meeting agendas, with regular daily viewing on school and government access channels. Even the US Congress and Supreme Court got into the act!

The ease, utility, and popularity of frequent daily exertion enforced by recess breaks set off a chain reaction. This really succeeded in driving public policy toward a societal restructuring to accommodate higher levels of physical activity.

Corporate and Nonprofit Workplaces

Changes radiated out from schools and other government health and human services agencies to small businesses and corporations, places of worship, hospitals and clinics, and other community institutions. Each type of organization brought its own opportunities for further dissemination through its professional networks.

The success of recess breaks in the public sector and early-adopter organizations in the private sector generated widespread media attention. This visibility finally convinced the bulk of private corporations (intermediate and late adopters) that it was in their own best interest to assume responsibility for their employees' health. The marketing *offer* was enhanced by research and practice demonstration of competitive advantages in terms of increased productivity, health care cost containment, tax incentives (for utilizing evidence-based interventions), and carbon footprint credits. Other advantages included bolstering their "green" credentials, making community benefit dollars also add to the bottom line in the case of health care organizations permitting a little legal "double-dipping," and improving the health and cognitive functioning of future employees. This resulted in a privatization of a large and important subset of chronic disease prevention and control, as the private sector is more adept at widespread and sustainable dissemination than the public sector.

The foundation for the tax incentives was provided by the extensive research by economists during the run-up to the 2010 census, especially those interested in labor and health, to define and quantify the difference between the cost to the consumer and the cost to society of certain health-compromising products. For example, society finally recognized and addressed the fact that 99¢ burgers were grossly underpriced because of government subsidies. They probably really cost society much more than salads, but salads at most fast food joints cost four times as much as burgers. Economists call this a market failure, or a failure of the free market to appropriately price commodities so that the seller and buyers bear all of the costs. The grounding of the numbers in reality garnered the support for the passage of consumption taxes to recoup government expenditures for inactivity-promoting products and services—cars, television, and movies, among them—expenditures that included higher charges for ambulance and emergency medical services, Medicare- and Medicaid-funded hospitalizations and ER visits, ICU days, surgeries (especially bariatric), long-term care provision, and rehabilitation services.

In particular, the corporate demand for training and assistance in implementing *Instant Recess* and other wellness policies and practices generated a flood of demand, a burgeoning market that shifted to the private sector, increasingly filled by private vendors that replaced universities and health departments. Vendors were contracted by self-insured corporations and insurance companies serving smaller businesses. These vendors and insurers represented a key mechanism for the dissemination of work-site wellness strategies within the private sector. Ever since wellness programs were required to adhere to standardized reporting of outcomes, the dismal success rates of even the best commercial weight loss programs were finally revealed: fewer than 1 percent of their clients and patients sustained clinically significant losses for 18 months or more. Employers realized and accepted the futility of weight loss and other individually focused education and counseling, and redirected their resources to changing their organizational culture and physical surroundings. Recess breaks then became a regular part of the benefits packages requested by unions and offered by human resource departments of progressive companies, with others following suit in short order.

Entertainment Media

We're still in the 2010s, but this next segment was easy to predict. *Instant Recess*, not surprisingly, supplied a bonanza of commercial opportunities for celebrities from Arnold Schwarzenegger to Tyra Banks. Packaging their own signature brief activity bouts in CD and DVD "star vehicles" proved to be quite palatable to actors, broadcast journalists, musicians, and other pop stars with corporate sponsorship and political sensitivities. Oprah Winfrey began hosting weekly *Instant Recess* breaks featuring a lineup of stars and fitness gurus, who used this as a tremendous marketing venue to launch their own 10-minute breaks.

A pivotal moment in taking *Instant Recess* to the next level was R&B singer and songwriter Usher's debut of his *Instant Recess* break at the halftime of an NFL game. Sponsored by a major insurance company and a large nonprofit managed care organization, the event packed the stadium and even the parking lots around the big-screen TVs. It drew a national TV audience of 10 million viewers, and the international audience was twice that. By showtime, the price of a thirty-second ad rivaled that of the Super Bowl. Usher's *Instant Recess* CD and DVD downloads raked in $20 million that night, and coattail sales of *Instant Recess* CDs and DVDs by other sports figures and entertainment celebs took several to the top of the Billboard chart. Professional sports teams' ringtone downloads alone produced revenues sufficient to underwrite their philanthropic initiatives promoting fitness.

In fact, in no small part due to Usher's support, recess breaks produced a resurgence of upbeat music videos with "dance moves for dummies" packaged in 5- to 10-minute segments. Prompting a feeding frenzy, these products were used in political meetings and on TV shows, downloaded by youth from iTunes and Amazon, posted on YouTube and Facebook, and spoofed on *Saturday Night Live* and late-night talk shows. They were also distributed by large corporations as a part of their wellness subcontractors' services, a burgeoning business outlet that expanded quickly, given the aging of the baby boomers and increased demand among people at increasingly higher risk for chronic disease at younger ages.

The hottest reality TV show became a kids' "Got Moves?" contest, a cross between the popular *Dancing with the Stars* and *American Idol*, sponsored by the Dairy Council's "Got Milk?" campaign, with the proviso that only low-fat milk or other nutrient-rich options could be advertised. This followed the runaway success of school district "Think Ya Got Moves?" competitions sponsored by sports teams. Winners of these competitions who maintained at least a B grade point average were featured during pregame and half-time recognition events doing their moves with celebs and the teams' players and cheerleaders. On occasion, their moves even made it into their favorite player's own *Instant Recess* break.

Society

People became increasingly intolerant of sitting for long intervals without moving around. Decreases in sedentariness and increases in physical activity across cities and counties and regions were captured in public health surveillance. Politicians were spurred to act, and act they did. Regulations imposed hefty fines on workplaces requiring extended sitting without interruption for activity. Laws were passed to place excise taxes on sedentary-promoting products, which subsidized tax breaks for organizations certified as "well workplaces." First-time heart attacks declined, dialysis units were shuttered, and emergency rooms were really slow—most were open only late at night and on weekends.

And *finally*, at long last, the political will emerged to create a built environment promoting physical activity and fitness. Public transit funding dominated transportation sector investment, choking off new highway construction and forcing the imposition of tolls to support basic maintenance. Gas taxes also had to be raised for road maintenance, as people became less and less willing to channel public funding into private transportation. The urban freeway was truly a thing of the past! Multilane high-speed roads became few and far between as high-speed trains diverted traffic from roads and customers from airplanes for regional routes. Historical preservation interests experienced a resurgence, which shrank city streets and restored village centers and brick lanes. As in Europe, most urban areas and even suburban villages became fairly densely populated—activity friendly for walking and biking, and restrictive and inhospitable for driving. Bike-exchange programs blanketed urban and suburban areas, even turning a profit that was used to lower the cost of bus and light-rail tickets for commuters. Passenger elevators were rarely included in buildings under five stories, saving costs that were plowed back into urban renewal, including green construction. Mixed-use designs became the rule, not the exception. Spurred by a coalition of activists working for environmental justice and against global climate change, low-income areas were also transformed, and economically driven residential segregation began to erode. The American carbon footprint plummeted. This provided the needed leverage to influence change throughout the developed and developing world by walking the talk and using American ingenuity to align economic, development, and environmental conservation.

TOWARD A BRIGHTER FUTURE . . .

Arresting the trends toward increasing sedentariness will require innovative, systemic change across many sectors of society. Leisure time activity alone, in the context of the ubiquitous social, cultural, and physical environmental drivers of sitting time, will clearly be insufficient to prevent chronic disease and to restore energy balance and the healthier, more stable weights of a half century ago (Owen, Bauman, and Brown 2009). Change approaches must build individual capability and organizational capacity for physical activity engagement, create new social norms, and transform the physical environment to support higher levels of energy expenditure population-wide.

There are signs of life. In 2009, ever-progressive New York City issued its first street-design manual, taking the guides issued in recent years in other cities like Chicago and San Francisco a step closer to formal policy adoption and implementation (Chen 2009). This was a culmination of two years of work led by their transportation department and involving more than a dozen other city agencies. The document reflects a vision of streets not merely as thoroughfares for cars, but as public spaces incorporating safety, aesthetics, and environmental and community concerns—a more activity-friendly place with neighborhood traffic circles, raised intersections, turnabouts, pedestrian "priority zones," and dedicated bike lanes sequestered from automobile traffic.

While all of this needs to happen, it can't all be done at once. That's where *Instant Recess* comes in. Public health professionals have labored long and hard to strategically focus on priorities, but progress has been slow and we need a catalyst. Recess is one of the few physical activity representations that resurrect for adults a time in life when the motivation to be active was inherent and irrepressible—before it was engineered out of us!

Momentum is building at the time of this writing. *Instant Recess* was featured in the national media a number of times during 2009 and early 2010. We have begun providing training, technical assistance, implementation support materials, and other resources to several agencies or networks at the state and national levels, including California's Women,

Infants, and Children (WIC) program, the California Department of Public Health's USDA-funded Network for a Healthy California, the California Center for Public Health Advocacy and California League of Cities' Healthy Eating Active Living (HEAL) Cities campaign, and the Minnesota state departments of parks and recreation, education, and health, in concert with a couple of the state's pro sports teams.

An unsolicited e-mail message in April 2010 to the state WIC program from Maureen Clark, one of the WIC agency directors, provided a vote of confidence:

> As a result of incorporating daily physical activity breaks and "lift-off" training, the corporate culture and work environment has dramatically changed at Community Resource Project, Inc. Comments such as, "That was fun" and "Let's do that again" are regularly heard in our office. We see more smiles and laughs during the day, and that has definitely improved staff morale and productivity while decreasing stress. We are grateful for . . . the "Lift-off" training, as it's helped reenergize us and recommit our efforts towards employee health and wellness.

And there's an opportunity for *Instant Recess* to regularly take to the national air waves. A seed grant from our CDC disparities center to the Washington, DC, public radio station WPFW to broadcast live *Instant Recess* breaks for simultaneous participation at community sites has led to an endorsement by the national Pacifica Network and a role for *Instant Recess* in bringing "boots on the ground" community engagement to the launch and implementation of the National Physical Activity Plan. Of course, my involvement with the first lady's campaign to end the childhood obesity epidemic is now affording me a level of visibility and credibility that I'm only beginning to fathom. After my appointment, my department chair, Fred Zimmerman, quipped tongue in cheek, "You spend the first twenty years of your career trying to get people to pay attention to you, and the second twenty years trying to get them to leave you alone."

Some people have argued that legislative policy precedes and drives norm change (Swinburn 2008). History suggests otherwise. The political will to drive legislation occurred late in the tobacco control movement, and it was dependent on preexisting social and cultural norm changes. California's smoke-free workplace act, passed in 1995 and implemented in 1998, was preceded by many years of organizationally imposed smoking bans and, subsequently, regulatory policies (including those required to receive federal funding) to maintain smoke-free workplaces. In other words, decisions by organizational leaders in different layers of society were the necessary and sufficient ingredient of change.

Barack Obama's election signaled, at least for a moment, a return of American optimism and collectivism, bringing with it an appreciation for and modeling of health and fitness at the highest level. So he hasn't quite quit smoking yet (at least as this book went to press). Nobody's perfect! And that's also the point. We can't pursue perfection at the expense of the good. We certainly don't want to decimate our future in those communities at high risk for chronic disease—who knows into what circumstances the next generation's visionary leaders will be born?

And I learned a long time ago from my mentor Les Breslow that real success is not about me—what I can do, how great I am—it's about influence. What can I inspire others to do? If we learned nothing else from the 2008 election, I hope we truly understand that the power to effect change is within our grasp.

I subscribe to the Margaret Mead school of thought—"Never doubt that a small group of thoughtful, committed citizens can change the world. Indeed, it is the *only* thing that ever has." And Gandhi's "You must be the change you wish to see in the world."

And, truly I am my father's child in terms of stubbornness and persistence. I've always embraced the Harriet Tubman "Make a way out of no way" approach. (The expression comes from my dear friend and creative collaborator Kim Jordan.) Tubman is one of my all-time *she-roes*, the historical leader most closely associated with the Underground Railroad, the patchwork of sympathetic abolitionists' homes, backwoods trails and paths, covert cultural communication signals such as drumming and gospel hymns, and displays of sheer cunning and determination in avoiding apprehension that helped many slaves escape the brutality of the "peculiar institution." I wrote "In My Father's House" on Independence Day in 1998, on the eve of the Interfaith Pilgrimage of the Middle

In My Father's House

I feel the
footsteps
Of our ancestors
Soles beating
Bodies heating
For a fleeting
Moment of
freedom

I hear the
drumbeats
Of our
predecessors
Voices roaring
Spirits soaring
Energies pouring
Out to the

courageous
I see the
movements
Of our
forefathers
Muscles gaining
Lungs straining
Perspiration raining
Long preparation

I know the
silences
Of our
foremothers
Lips shushing
Feet rushing
Faces flushing

Path to freedom
I taste the hunger
Of our forebears
Stomachs grumbling
Whispers rumbling
Thoughts stumbling
Settle only for
freedom
Poised to live
Prepared to die

Knowing the truth
Shedding the lie

Making a way
For *us* to fly!

T___' *(July 4, 1998)*

Passage—a healing journey of a tour group of African Americans and whites that started in Richmond, Virginia, by walking the path along the James River from the slave ships to the auction block. Todd Berrien and I participated in this march, and it was powerful and spiritually moving. The group made other historical stops, ending at the West African British, Dutch, and Portuguese seaports where our ancestors were sold into slavery.

In fact, if I ever have the philanthropic wherewithal, I'm going to seize that $40 million naming opportunity to establish the Harriet Ross Tubman School of Public Health at UCLA.

I'll leave you with one more poem for the road.

Wilma Rudolph's Legacy

Wilma died yesterday.
And I never knew her.
Long and lanky like me.
Never had a chance to meet her.
But I knew her spirit
Because it was ours . . .

Wilma died yesterday.
She shared a name with _my_ Wilma.
The "Fonzie" of the neighborhood.
Feared, respected and worshipped.
The speediest kid on the block
Whose physical prowess was
     legendary.
The girl with the legs of a stallion
Voted the brickhouse of West
     Jr. High.
My childhood she-roe.

Wilma died yesterday.
To me, she embodied greatness.
"Physical fitness," echoing JFK,
"The basis of _all_ other forms of
     excellence."
She and Shirley and Barbara and
     Audre . . .
And my renegade aunts
Were _my_ role models.
_My_ substance of things hoped for.
_My_ evidence of things not seen.
They worked twice as hard.
Were twice as good.
Survived, succeeded, thrived,
     flourished.

Lived their dreams and, in so doing,
Sowed the seeds for mine.
Because of them, formidable odds
     against me
Weren't part of _my_ equation.
Were a challenge, not an obstacle.
They kept my hope alive
And, in times of despair,
Rekindled it
When the last embers had ceased to
     glow.

Wilma died yesterday.
She and the others are deceased
Or diseased.
Too young.
Too soon.
But their drive spurs my ambition.
Their spirits fuel my passion.
And I owe them
Social justice.
Collective empowerment.
A truly free society
Guaranteeing each child
A clean and safe environment,
Quality health care and
Excellent public education.
The realization of equal access to
     opportunity.
I owe them the assurance that the
     torch
Has indeed been passed.

                    T___· (November 13, 1994)

References

Appendices are available at www.toniyancey.com.

Aldana, S. G. 2001. Financial impact of health promotion programs: A comprehensive review of the literature. *Am J Health Promot* 15 (5):296–320.

Andersen, R. E., S. C. Franckowiak, J. Snyder, S. J. Bartlett, and K. R. Fontaine. 1998. Can inexpensive signs encourage the use of stairs? Results from a community intervention. *Ann Intern Med* 129 (5):363–9.

Andersen, R. E., S. C. Franckowiak, K. B. Zuzak, E. S. Cummings, S. J. Bartlett, and C. J. Crespo. 2006. Effects of a culturally sensitive sign on the use of stairs in African American commuters. *Soz Praventivmed* 51 (6):373–80.

Anderson, L. H., B. C. Martinson, A. L. Crain, N. P. Pronk, R. R. Whitebird, P. J. O'Connor, and L. J. Fine. 2005. Health care charges associated with physical inactivity, overweight, and obesity. *Prev Chronic Dis* 2 (4):A09.

Andreasen, Alan R. 1995. *Marketing social change changing behavior to promote health, social development, and the environment.* San Francisco: Jossey-Bass.

Andreyeva, T., and R. Sturm. 2006. Physical activity and changes in health care costs in late middle age. *J Phys Act Health* 3:S6–S19.

Babey, S. H., A. L. Diamant, E. R. Brown, and T. Hastert. 2005. California adolescents increasingly inactive. Policy Brief. *UCLA Cent Health Policy Res* (PB2005-3):1–7.

Bandura, A. 1989. Human agency in social cognitive theory. *Am Psychol* 44 (9):1175–84.

———. 2004. Health promotion by social cognitive means. *Health Educ Behav* 31 (2):143–64.

BBC News. 2009. Philippine jailhouse rocks to Thriller. Available at: http://news.bbc.co.uk/2/hi/asia-pacific/6917318.stm. July 26.

Bellisari, A. 2008. Evolutionary origins of obesity. *Obes Rev* 9 (2):165–80.

Besser, L. M., and A. L. Dannenberg. 2005. Walking to public transit: Steps to help meet physical activity recommendations. *Am J Prev Med* 29 (4):273–80.

Blair, S. N., H. W. Kohl 3rd, C. E. Barlow, R. S. Paffenbarger Jr., L. W. Gibbons, and C. A. Macera. 1995. Changes in physical fitness and all-cause mortality: A prospective study of healthy and unhealthy men. *JAMA* 273 (14):1093–8.

Bland, P. C., L. An, S. S. Foldes, N. Garrett, and N. L. Alesci. 2009. Modifiable health behaviors and short-term medical costs among health plan members. *Am J Health Promot* 23 (4):265–73.

Boarnet, M. G., C. L. Anderson, K. Day, T. McMillan, and M. Alfonzo. 2005. Evaluation of the California Safe Routes to School legislation: Urban form changes and children's active transportation to school. *Am J Prev Med* 28 (2 Suppl 2):134–40.

Breslow, L., and N. Breslow. 1993. Health practices and disability: Some evidence from Alameda County. *Prev Med* 22 (1):86–95.

Brown, W. J., A. E. Bauman, and N. Owen. 2009. Stand up, sit down, keep moving: Turning circles in physical activity research? *Br J Sports Med* 43 (2):86–8.

Brownson, R. C., T. K. Boehmer, and D. A. Luke. 2005. Declining rates of physical activity in the United States: What are the contributors? *Annu Rev Public Health* 26:421–43.

Bryant, Julie. 2001. Fat is a $34 billion business. *Atlanta Business Chronicle*, Sep 21.

Bull, F. C., T. Armstrong, T. Dixon, S. A. Ham, A. Neiman, and M. Pratt. 2003. Burden attributable to physical inactivity: Examination of the 2002 World Health Report estimates. *Med Sci Sports Exerc* 35 (5 [Suppl 1]):S359.

California Nutrition Network and California Department of Health Service. 2004. Workplace nutrition and physical activity. *Issue Brief 1* (1):1–8.

Camerer, C. 1999. Behavioral economics: Reunifying psychology and economics. *Proc Natl Acad Sci USA* 96 (19):10575–7.

Carter, J. B., and E. W. Banister. 1994. Musculoskeletal problems in VDT work: A review. *Ergonomics* 37:1623–48. Quoted in Galinsky, T. et al. 2007, 520. Supplementary breaks and stretching exercises for data entry operators: A follow-up field study. *Am J Ind Med* 50 (7):519–27.

Center for Responsive Politics. 2008. Food and beverage and food processing and sales industry categories. Available from http://www.opensecrets.org/industries/indus.php?ind=A09.

Chen, D. W. 2009. In the future, the city's streets are to behave. *New York Times*, May 20, A23.

Chenoweth, D. 2005. The economic costs of physical inactivity, obesity, and overweight in California adults: Health care, workers' compensation, and lost productivity. Sacramento, CA: California Department of Health Services.

Church, T. S., J. L. Kuk, R. Ross, E. L. Priest, E. Biltoft, and S. N. Blair. 2006. Association of cardiorespiratory fitness, body mass index, and waist circumference to nonalcoholic fatty liver disease. *Gastroenterology* 130 (7):2023–30.

Colditz, G. A. 1999. Economic costs of obesity and inactivity. *Med Sci Sports Exerc* 31 (11 Suppl):S663–7.

Cooper, Ken. 1970. *The new aerobics*. New York: M. Evans.

Costanza, M. C., S. Beer-Borst, and A. Morabia. 2007. Achieving energy balance at the population level through increases in physical activity. *Am J Public Health* 97 (3):520–5.

Crawford, P. B., W. Gosliner, P. Strode, S. E. Samuels, C. Burnett, L. Craypo, and A. K. Yancey. 2004. Walking the talk: Fit WIC wellness programs improve self-efficacy in pediatric obesity prevention counseling. *Am J Public Health* 94 (9):1480–5.

Cummings, P., F. P. Rivara, C. M. Olson, and K. M. Smith. 2006. Changes in traffic crash mortality rates attributed to use of alcohol, or lack of a seat belt, air bag, motorcycle helmet, or bicycle helmet, United States, 1982–2001. *Inj Prev* 12 (3):148–54.

Das, Andrew. 2009. More Wii warriors are playing hurt. *New York Times*, April 20, D5.

de Jong, J., K. A. Lemmink, M. Stevens, M. H. de Greef, P. Rispens, A. C. King, and T. Mulder. 2006. Six-month effects of the Groningen active living model (GALM) on physical activity, health and fitness outcomes in sedentary and underactive older adults aged 55–65. *Patient Educ Couns* 62 (1):132–41.

Donnelly, J. E., J. L. Greene, C. A. Gibson, R. A. Washburn, D. K. Sullivan, K. D. DuBose, M. S. Mayo, K. H. Schmelzle, J. J. Ryan, S. L. Williams, D. J. Jacobsen, and B. Smith. 2009. Physical Activity Across the Curriculum (PAAC): A randomized, controlled trial to promote physical activity and diminish overweight and obesity in elementary school children. *Prev Med* 49:336–41.

Dorfman, L., and L. Wallack. 2007. Moving nutrition upstream: The case for reframing obesity. *J Nutr Educ Behav* 39 (2 Suppl):S45–S50.

Dorfman, L., and A. K. Yancey. 2009. Promoting physical activity and healthy eating: Convergence in framing the role of industry. *Prev Med* 49:303–5.

Eaton, S. B., B. I. Strassman, R. M. Nesse, J. V. Neel, P. W. Ewald, G. C. Williams, A. B. Weder, S. B. Eaton 3rd, S. Lindeberg, M. J. Konner, I. Mysterud, and L. Cordain. 2002. Evolutionary health promotion. *Prev Med* 34 (2):109–18.

Ekkekakis, P., E. Lind, and S. Vazou. 2009. Affective responses to increasing levels of exercise intensity in normal-weight, overweight, and obese middle-aged women. *Obesity* 18 (1):79–85.

Fenton, M. 2009. Physical activity in the US: The urgency of change. Paper read at National Physical Activity Plan Conference, July 1, 2009, Washington, DC.

Finkelstein, E. A., J. G. Trogdon, J. W. Cohen, and W. Dietz. 2009. Annual medical spending attributable to obesity: Payer- and service-specific estimates. *Health Aff* 28(5):w822–31.

Flegal, K. M., M. D. Carroll, C. L. Ogden, and C. L. Johnson. 2002. Prevalence and trends in obesity among US adults, 1999–2000. *JAMA* 288 (14):1723–7.

Foerster, S. B., K. W. Kizer, L. K. Disogra, D. G. Bal, B. F. Krieg, and K. L. Bunch. 1995. California's "5 a day—for better health!" campaign: An innovative population-based effort to effect large-scale dietary change. *Am J Prev Med* 11 (2):124–31.

Freedman, D. S., L. K. Khan, M. K. Serdula, C. L. Ogden, and W. H. Dietz. 2006. Racial and ethnic differences in secular trends for childhood BMI, weight, and height. *Obesity* 14 (2):301–8.

French, S. A., M. Story, and R. W. Jeffery. 2001. Environmental influences on eating and physical activity. *Annu Rev Public Health* 22:309–35.

Friedman, Thomas L. 2008. *Hot, flat, and crowded: Why we need a green revolution, and how it can renew America.* New York: Farrar, Straus and Giroux.

Fuemmeler, B. F., C. Baffi, L. C. Masse, A. A. Atienza, and W. D. Evans. 2007. Employer and healthcare policy interventions aimed at adult obesity. *Am J Prev Med* 32 (1):44–51.

Galinsky, T., N. Swanson, S. Sauter, R. Dunkin, J. Hurrell, and L. Schleifer. 2007. Supplementary breaks and stretching exercises for data entry operators: A follow-up field study. *Am J Ind Med* 50 (7):519–27.

Georgeson, M., L. E. Thorpe, M. Merlino, T. R. Frieden, and J. E. Fielding. 2005. Shortchanged? An assessment of chronic disease programming in major US city health departments. *J Urban Health* 82 (2):183–90.

Gibson, C. A., B. K. Smith, K. D. DuBose, J. L. Greene, B. W. Bailey, S. L. Williams, J. J. Ryan, K. H. Schmelzle, R. A. Washburn, D. K. Sullivan, M. S. Mayo, and J. E. Donnelly. 2008. Physical activity across the curriculum: Year one process evaluation results. *Int J Behav Nutr Phys Act* 5:36.

Goetzel, R. Z. 2009. Do prevention or treatment services save money? The wrong debate. *Health Aff* 28 (1):37–41.

Grier, S., and C. A. Bryant. 2005. Social marketing in public health. *Annu Rev Public Health* 26:319–39.

Haapanen-Niemi, N., S. Miilunpalo, M. Pasanen, I. Vuori, P. Oja, and J. Malmberg. 2000. Body mass index, physical inactivity and low level of physical fitness as determinants of all-cause and cardiovascular disease mortality: 16 y follow-up of middle-aged and elderly men and women. *Int J Obes Relat Metab Disord* 24 (11):1465–74.

Halbfinger, D. M. 2009. Corzine points a spotlight at his rival's waistline. *New York Times*, Oct 8, A27.

Hamilton, M. T., D. G. Hamilton, and T. W. Zderic. 2007. Role of low energy expenditure and sitting in obesity, metabolic syndrome, type 2 diabetes, and cardiovascular disease. *Diabetes* 56 (11):2655–67.

Hamilton, M. T., G. N. Healy, D. W. Dunstan, T. W. Zderic, and N. Owen. 2008. Too little exercise and too much sitting: Inactivity physiology and the need for new recommendations on sedentary behavior. *Curr Cardiovasc Risk Rep* 2:292–298.

Hawley, J. A., and J. O. Holloszy. 2009. Exercise: It's the real thing! *Nutr Rev* 67 (3):172–8.

Hickey, G. Dressing, dribbling and now directing. *Richmond Times Dispatch*. July 14, 1996, B1.

Honas, J. J., R. A. Washburn, B. K. Smith, J. L. Greene, and J. E. Donnelly. 2008. Energy expenditure of the physical activity across the curriculum intervention. *Med Sci Sports Exerc* 40 (8):1501–5.

Hu, F. B., T. Y. Li, G. A. Colditz, W. C. Willett, and J. E. Manson. 2003. Television watching and other sedentary behaviors in relation to risk of obesity and type 2 diabetes mellitus in women. *JAMA* 289 (14):1785–91.

Huhman, M., C. Heitzler, and F. Wong. 2004. The VERB campaign logic model: A tool for planning and evaluation. *Prev Chronic Dis* 1 (3):A11.

Institute of Medicine of the National Academies, Committee on Food Marketing and the Diets of Children and Youth. 2006. *Food marketing to children and youth: Threat or opportunity?* Eds. J. Michael McGinnis, Jennifer Appleton Gootman, and Vivica I. Kraak. Washington, DC: National Academies Press.

James, S. A., L. Jamjoum, T. E. Raghunathan, D. S. Strogatz, E. D. Furth, and P. G. Khazanie. 1998. Physical activity and NIDDM in African-Americans. The Pitt County Study. *Diabetes Care* 21 (4):555–62.

Katz, M. 2009. Tossing out the diet and embracing the fat. *New York Times*, July 16, E3.

Katzmarzyk, P. T., and C. Mason. 2009. The physical activity transition. *J Phys Act Health* 6 (3):269–80.

Kaufman, Francine Ratner. 2005. *Diabesity: The obesity-diabetes epidemic that threatens America—and what we must do to stop it.* New York: Bantam Books.

Keeler, E. B., W. G. Manning, J. P. Newhouse, E. M. Sloss, and J. Wasserman.

1989. The external costs of a sedentary life-style. *Am J Public Health* 79 (8):975–81.

Kersh, R., and J. Morone. 2002. The politics of obesity: Seven steps to government action. *Health Aff* 21 (6):142–53.

Kessel, W., C. Beato, and P. Royall. 2004. Overweight and obesity in America. Los Angeles: Paper presented at the Region IX Obesity Meeting. September 18.

Kessler, David A. 2009. *The end of overeating: Taking control of the insatiable American appetite*. Emmaus, PA: Rodale.

King, A. C., R. F. Oman, G. S. Brassington, D. L. Bliwise, and W. L. Haskell. 1997. Moderate-intensity exercise and self-rated quality of sleep in older adults: A randomized controlled trial. *JAMA* 277 (1):32–7.

Lakdawalla, D., J. Bhattacharya, and D. P. Goldman. 2004. Are the young becoming more disabled? *Health Aff* 23 (1):168–176.

Landsberg, L. 2008. Body fat distribution and cardiovascular risk: A tale of 2 sites. *Arch Intern Med* 168 (15):1607–8.

Lara, A., A. K. Yancey, R. Tapia-Conye, Y. Flores, P. Kuri-Morales, R. Mistry, E. Subirats, and W. J. McCarthy. 2008. Pausa para tu salud: Reduction of weight and waistlines by integrating exercise breaks into workplace organizational routine. *Prev Chronic Dis* 5 (1):A12.

Lawrence, A., L. Lewis, G. J. Hofmeyr, T. Dowswell, and C. Styles. 2009. Maternal positions and mobility during first stage labour. *Cochrane Database Syst Rev* (2):CD003934.

Lee, I. M., R. Ewing, and H. D. Sesso. 2009. The built environment and physical activity levels: The Harvard Alumni Health Study. *Am J Prev Med* 37 (4):293–8.

Leslie, J., A. Yancey, W. McCarthy, S. Albert, C. Wert, O. Miles, and J. James. 1999. Development and implementation of a school-based nutrition and fitness promotion program for ethnically diverse middle-school girls. *J Am Diet Assoc* 99 (8):967–70.

Levine, J. A., S. K. McCrady, L. M. Lanningham-Foster, P. H. Kane, R. C. Foster, and C. U. Manohar. 2008. The role of free-living daily walking in human weight gain and obesity. *Diabetes* 57 (3):548–54.

Levine, J. A., and J. M. Miller. 2007. The energy expenditure of using a "walk-and-work" desk for office workers with obesity. *Br J Sports Med* 41 (9):558–61.

Levine, James, and Selene Yeager. 2009. *Move a little, lose a lot: New NEAT science reveals how to be thinner, happier, and smarter*. New York: Crown.

Libby, P. 2005. The forgotten majority: Unfinished business in cardiovascular risk reduction. *J Am Coll Cardiol* 46 (7):1225–8.

Lynch, K. B., C. B. Corbin, and C. L. Sidman. 2009. Testing compensation: Does recreational basketball impact adult activity levels? *J Phys Act Health* 6 (3):321–6.

Mahar, M. T., S. K. Murphy, D. A. Rowe, J. Golden, A. T. Shields, and T. D. Raedeke. 2006. Effects of a classroom-based program on physical activity and on-task behavior. *Med Sci Sports Exerc* 38 (12):2086–94.

Mann, T., A. J. Tomiyama, E. Westling, A. M. Lew, B. Samuels, and J. Chatman. 2007. Medicare's search for effective obesity treatments: Diets are not the answer. *Am Psychol* 62 (3):220–33.

Mark, A. E., and I. Janssen. 2009. Influence of bouts of physical activity on overweight in youth. *Am J Prev Med* 36 (5):416–21.

Maugham, W. Somerset. 1943. *The Razor's Edge*. New York: Doubleday.

Medina, John J. 2008. *Brain rules: 12 principles for surviving and thriving at work, home, and school*. Seattle: Pear.

Messer, K., J. P. Pierce, S. H. Zhu, A. M. Hartman, W. K. Al-Delaimy, D. R. Trinidad, and E. A. Gilpin. 2007. The California Tobacco Control Program's effect on adult smokers: (1) Smoking cessation. *Tob Control* 16 (2):85–90.

Miyashita, M., S. F. Burns, and D. J. Stensel. 2006. Exercise and postprandial lipemia: Effect of continuous compared with intermittent activity patterns. *Am J Clin Nutr* 83 (1):24–9.

Mokdad, A. H., J. S. Marks, D. F. Stroup, and J. L. Gerberding. 2004. Actual causes of death in the United States, 2000. *JAMA* 291 (10):1238–45.

Morabia, A., and M. C. Costanza. 2009. Active encouragement of physical activity during school recess. *Prev Med* 48 (4):305–6.

Murray, N. 2009. Pass & Catch. Paper read at Institute of Medicine Standing Committee on Childhood Obesity Prevention, February 5, in Austin, TX.

Narayan, K. M., J. P. Boyle, T. J. Thompson, S. W. Sorensen, and D. F. Williamson. 2003. Lifetime risk for diabetes mellitus in the United States. *JAMA* 290 (14):1884–90.

National Diabetes Education Program. 2007. Diabetes at Work Workshop Kit. Available at www.ndep.nih.gov/resources/business.htm. Washington, DC: National Diabetes Education Program.

National Women's Law Center and Harvard School of Public Health. 2004. *Keeping score: Girls' participation in high school athletics in Massachusetts*. Ed. Harvard School of Public Health. Boston: Harvard University. Available from http://www.hsph.harvard.edu/press/releases/sports/keepingscore report.pdf.

Neighmond, P. 2009. Expert: 10-minute workouts can have big payoff. National Public Radio. Broadcast February 26. Available at http://m.npr.org/news/front/101151713.

Oberlander, J. B., and B. Lyons. 2009. Beyond incrementalism? SCHIP and the politics of health reform. *Health Aff* 28 (3):w399–410.

Ogden, C. L., M. D. Carroll, L. R. Curtin, M. A. McDowell, C. J. Tabak, and K. M. Flegal. 2006. Prevalence of overweight and obesity in the United States, 1999–2004. *JAMA* 295 (13):1549–55.

Olshansky, S. J., D. J. Passaro, R. C. Hershow, J. Layden, B. A. Carnes, J. Brody, L. Hayflick, R. N. Butler, D. B. Allison, and D. S. Ludwig. 2005. A potential decline in life expectancy in the United States in the 21st century. *N Engl J Med* 352 (11):1138–45.

Owen, N., A. Bauman, and W. Brown. 2009. Too much sitting: A novel and important predictor of chronic disease risk? *Br J Sports Med* 43 (2):81–3.

Passe, D. H., M. Horn, and R. Murray. 2000. Impact of beverage acceptability on fluid intake during exercise. *Appetite* 35 (3):219–29.

Pearson, S. D., and S. R. Lieber. 2009. Financial penalties for the unhealthy? Ethical guidelines for holding employees responsible for their health. *Health Aff* 28 (3):845–52.

Pescatello, L. S., and J. L. VanHeest. 2000. Physical activity mediates a healthier body weight in the presence of obesity. *Br J Sports Med* 34 (2):86–93.

Physical Activity Guidelines Advisory Committee. 2008. Physical Activity Guidelines Advisory Committee Report, 2008. Washington, DC: US Department of Health and Human Services. Available at http://www.health.gov/paguidelines/committeereport.aspx. Accessed October 7, 2008.

Pollan, Michael. 2006. *The omnivore's dilemma: A natural history of four meals.* New York: Penguin.

Pronk, N. P., M. J. Goodman, P. J. O'Connor, and B. C. Martinson. 1999. Relationship between modifiable health risks and short-term health care charges. *JAMA* 282 (23):2235–9.

Pronk, S. J., N. P. Pronk, A. Sisco, D. S. Ingalls, and C. Ochoa. 1995. Impact of a daily 10-minute strength and flexibility program in a manufacturing plant. *Am J Health Promot* 9 (3):175–8.

Ratey, J. J., and E. Hagerman. 2008. *Spark: The revolutionary new science of exercise and the brain.* New York: Little, Brown.

Reaven, G. M. 1999. Insulin resistance: A chicken that has come to roost. *Ann N Y Acad Sci* 892:45–57.

Resnicow, K., A. Jackson, D. Blissett, T. Wang, F. McCarty, S. Rahotep, and S. Periasamy. 2005. Results of the healthy body healthy spirit trial. *Health Psychol* 24 (4):339–48.

Reuters. 2010. Routine "recess" a hit at White House obesity summit. April 9. Available at http://www.reuters.com/article/idUSTRE63900W20100410.

Rogers, Everett M. 2003. *Diffusion of innovations.* 5th ed. New York: Free Press.

Rowland, N. E., C. H. Vaughan, C. M. Mathes, and A. Mitra. 2008. Feeding behavior, obesity, and neuroeconomics. *Physiol Behav* 93 (1–2):97–109.

Schwimmer, J. B., T. M. Burwinkle, and J. W. Varni. 2003. Health-related quality of life of severely obese children and adolescents. *JAMA* 289 (14):1813–9.

Sibley, B. A., R. M. Ward, T. S. Yazvac, K. Zullig, and J. A. Potteiger. 2008. Making the grade with diet and exercise. *AASA Journal of Scholarship and Practice* 5 (2):38–45.

Simon, E. 2006. Companies are promoting better lifestyles. Associated Press, December 6.

Slusser, W. M., W. G. Cumberland, B. L. Browdy, D. M. Winham, and C. G. Neumann. 2005. Overweight in urban, low-income, African American and Hispanic children attending Los Angeles elementary schools: Research stimulating action. *Public Health Nutr* 8 (2):141–8.

Stefan, N., K. Kantartzis, J. Machann, F. Schick, C. Thamer, K. Rittig, B. Balletshofer, F. Machicao, A. Fritsche, and H. U. Haring. 2008. Identification and characterization of metabolically benign obesity in humans. *Arch Intern Med* 168 (15):1609–16.

Stewart, J. A., D. A. Dennison, H. W. Kohl, and J. A. Doyle. 2004. Exercise level and energy expenditure in the TAKE 10! in-class physical activity program. *J Sch Health* 74 (10):397–400.

Sturm, R. 2002. The effects of obesity, smoking, and drinking on medical problems and costs: Obesity outranks both smoking and drinking in its deleterious effects on health and health costs. *Health Aff* 21 (2):245–53.

———. 2004. The economics of physical activity: Societal trends and rationales for interventions. *Am J Prev Med* 27 (3 Suppl):126–35.

———. 2008. Stemming the global obesity epidemic: What can we learn from data about social and economic trends? *Public Health* 122 (8):739–46.

Swinburn, B. A. 2008. Obesity prevention: The role of policies, laws and regulations. *Aust New Zealand Health Policy* 5:12.

Taylor, W. C., A. K. Yancey, J. Leslie, N. G. Murray, S. S. Cummings, S. A. Sharkey, C. Wert, J. James, O. Miles, and W. J. McCarthy. 1999. Physical activity among African American and Latino middle school girls: Consistent beliefs, expectations, and experiences across two sites. *Women Health* 30 (2):67–82.

Thaler, Richard H., and Cass R. Sunstein. 2008. *Nudge: Improving decisions about health, wealth, and happiness.* New Haven, CT: Yale University Press.

Thomas, Katie. 2009. Left behind: A city team's struggle shows disparity in girls' sports. *New York Times*, June 14, A1.

Timperio, A., D. Cameron-Smith, C. Burns, and D. Crawford. 2000. The public's response to the obesity epidemic in Australia: Weight concerns and weight control practices of men and women. *Public Health Nutr* 3 (4):417–24.

Tirodkar, M. A., and A. Jain. 2003. Food messages on African American television shows. *Am J Public Health* 93 (3):439–41.

Troiano, R. P., D. Berrigan, K. W. Dodd, L. C. Masse, T. Tilert, and M. McDowell. 2008. Physical activity in the United States measured by accelerometer. *Med Sci Sports Exerc* 40 (1):181–8.

Trost, S. G. 2004. School physical education in the post-report era: An analysis from public health. *Journal of Teaching in Physical Education* 23:216–35.

———. 2007. Active education: Physical education, physical activity and academic performance. A research brief prepared for Active Living Research. Available at http://www.activelivingresearch.org/files/Active_Ed.pdf.

Truong, K. D., and R. Sturm. 2005. Weight gain trends across sociodemographic groups in the United States. *Am J Public Health* 95 (9):1602–6.

UCLA Center to Eliminate Health Disparities and Samuels & Associates. January 2007. *Failing Fitness: Physical Activity and Physical Education in Schools.* Funded by the California Endowment. Los Angeles. Available at http://www.calendow.org.

UCLA School of Public Health. 2003. Health Impact Assessment (HIA). Los Angeles: Partnership for Prevention and UCLA School of Public Health. Available from http://www.ph.ucla.edu/hs/health-impact/index.htm.

US Centers for Disease Control and Prevention. 2007. KidsWalk-to-School. Available at: http://www.cdc.gov/nccdphp/dnpa/kidswalk. Accessed May 11, 2009.

US Department of Health and Human Services. 2001. The surgeon general's call to action to prevent and decrease overweight and obesity. Washington DC: Public Health Service, Office of the Surgeon General.

Valente, T. W., S. Murphy, G. Huang, J. Gusek, J. Greene, and V. Beck. 2007. Evaluating a minor storyline on *ER* about teen obesity, hypertension, and 5 A Day. *J Health Commun* 12 (6):551–66.

Vigorous physical activity among high school students—United States, 1990. 1992. *MMWR Morb Mortal Wkly Rep* 41 (3):33–5.

Wang, F., T. McDonald, L. J. Champagne, and D. W. Edington. 2004. Relationship of body mass index and physical activity to health care costs among employees. *J Occup Environ Med* 46 (5):428–36.

Wang, Y., and T. Lobstein. 2006. Worldwide trends in childhood overweight and obesity. *Int J Pediatr Obes* 1 (1):11–25.

Weiner, J. 2004. Celebrating women's sports, one image at a time. *New York Times*, June 6, C6.

Westerterp-Plantenga, M. S., C. R. Verwegen, M. J. Ijedema, N. E. Wijckmans, and W. H. Saris. 1997. Acute effects of exercise or sauna on appetite in obese and nonobese men. *Physiol Behav* 62 (6):1345–54.

Willett, W. C. 2006. Trans fatty acids and cardiovascular disease: Epidemiological data. *Atheroscler Suppl* 7 (2):5–8.

Williams, C. L., B. J. Carter, D. L. Kibbe, and D. Dennison. 2009. Increasing physical activity in preschool: A pilot study to evaluate animal trackers. *J Nutr Educ Behav* 41 (1):47–52.

Wolin, K. Y., Y. Yan, G. A. Colditz, and I. M. Lee. 2009. Physical activity and colon cancer prevention: A meta-analysis. *Br J Cancer* 100 (4):611–6.

Yancey, A. K. 1997. Sports are good for girls. *Richmond Times-Dispatch*, May 12, A9.

————. 2009. The meta-volition model: Organizational leadership is the key ingredient in getting society moving, literally! *Prev Med* 49:342–51.

Yancey, A. K., B. L. Cole, R. Brown, J. D. Williams, A. Hillier, R. S. Kline, M. Ashe, S. A. Grier, D. Backman, and W. J. McCarthy. 2009. A cross-sectional prevalence study of ethnically targeted and general audience outdoor obesity-related advertising. *Milbank Q* 87 (1):155–84.

Yancey, A. K., J. E. Fielding, G. R. Flores, J. F. Sallis, W. J. McCarthy, and L. Breslow. 2007. Creating a robust public health infrastructure for physical activity promotion. *Am J Prev Med* 32 (1):68–78.

Yancey, A. K., D. Grant, S. Witt, N. Kravitz-Wirtz, and R. Mistry. 2010 (forthcoming). Role modeling, risk and resilience in California adolescents. *J Adolesc Health*.

Yancey, A. K., A. Jordan, J. Bradford, J. Voas, T. Eller, M. Buzzard, M. Welch, and W. McCarthy. 2003. Engaging high-risk populations in community-level fitness promotion: ROCK! Richmond. *Health Promotion Practice* 4 (2):180–8.

Yancey, A. K., L. B. Lewis, J. J. Guinyard, D. C. Sloan, L. M. Nascimento, L. Galloway-Gilliam, A. Diamant, and W. J. McCarthy. 2006. Putting promotion into practice: The African Americans Building a Legacy of Health organizational wellness program. *Health Promotion Practice* 7(3):233S–246S.

Yancey A. K., L. B. Lewis, D. C. Sloane, J. J. Guinyard, A. L. Diamant, L. M. Nascimento, W. J. McCarthy, and REACH Coalition. 2004. Leading by example: Process evaluation of a local health department-community collaboration to change organizational practice to incorporate physical activity. *J Public Health Manag Prac* 10(2):116–23.

Yancey, A. K., W. J. McCarthy, G. G. Harrison, W. K. Wong, J. M. Siegel, and J. Leslie. 2006. Challenges in improving fitness: Results of a community-based, randomized, controlled lifestyle change intervention. *J Womens Health* 15 (4):412–29.

Yancey, A. K., O. Miles, and A. Jordan. 1999. Organizational characteristics facilitating initiation and institutionalization of physical activity programs in a multi-ethnic, urban community. *Journal of Health Education* 30 (2):S44–S51.

Yancey, A. K., O. L. Miles, W. J. McCarthy, G. Sandoval, J. Hill, J. J. Leslie, and G. G. Harrison. 2001. Differential response to targeted recruitment strategies to fitness promotion research by African-American women of varying body mass index. *Ethn Dis* 11 (1):115–23.

Yancey, A. K., N. P. Pronk, and B. L. Cole. 2007. Workplace approaches to obesity prevention. In *Handbook of obesity prevention: A resource for health professionals*. Eds. S. K. Kumanyika and R. C. Brownson. New York: Springer.

Yancey, A. K., J. M. Siegel, and K. L. McDaniel. 2002. Role models, ethnic identity, and health-risk behaviors in urban adolescents. *Arch Pediatr Adolesc Med* 156 (1):55–61.

Yancey, A. K., P. A. Simon, W. J. McCarthy, A. S. Lightstone, and J.E. Fielding. Ethnic and gender differences in overweight self-perception: relationship to sedentariness. *Obes* 2006; 14: 980–8.

Yancey, A. K., C. M. Wold, W. J. McCarthy, M. D. Weber, B. Lee, P. A. Simon, and J. E. Fielding. 2004. Physical inactivity and overweight among Los Angeles County adults. *Am J Prev Med* 27 (2):146–52.

Yancey, Antronette K., Roshan Bastani, and Beth Glenn. 2007. Racial/ethnic disparities in health status. In *Changing the U.S. health care system: Key issues in health services, policy, and management*. Eds. R. Andersen, T. H. Rice, and G. F. Kominski. San Francisco: Jossey-Bass.

Zernike, K. 2003. Fight against fat shifting to the workplace. *New York Times*, Oct 12, A1.

About the Author

Toni (Antronette K.) Yancey, MD, MPH, is currently a professor in the Department of Health Services, UCLA School of Public Health, and is co-director of the UCLA Kaiser Permanente Center for Health Equity. Her primary research interests are in chronic disease prevention and adolescent health promotion. She returned to academia full time in 2001 after five years in public health practice, first as director of public health for the city of Richmond, Virginia, and then as director of chronic disease prevention and health promotion, Los Angeles County Department of Health Services. Dr. Yancey has authored more than a hundred twenty-five scientific publications, including briefs, book chapters, health promotion videos, and among those, more than eighty peer-reviewed journal articles and editorials. She has generated more than $30 million in extramural funds over the course of her career. She

253

serves on the Institute of Medicine Standing Committee on Childhood Obesity Prevention and the National Physical Activity Plan Coordinating Committee. She is the immediate past chair of the board of directors of the Oakland, California–based Public Health Institute. Dr. Yancey was recently appointed to the nine-member board of directors of the Partnership for a Healthier America, the nonprofit foundation supporting first lady Michelle Obama's Let's Move initiative, and the board of directors of Skokie, Illinois–based Action for Healthy Kids.

Dr. Yancey completed her undergraduate studies in biochemistry and molecular biology at Northwestern University, her medical degree and internship in psychiatry at Duke, and her preventive medicine residency/MPH at UCLA. She also practiced medicine and modeled professionally in New York City for five years after leaving her psychiatric residency. She is a basketball enthusiast and a poet/spoken word artist published in medical journals, including *Preventive Medicine* and the *American Journal of Preventive Medicine*, as well as several newspapers. Her book of poetry and art, a collaboration with artist Todd Berrien, *An Old Soul with a Young Spirit: Poetry in the Era of Desegregation Recovery*, was published in 1997 and sold out of its first printing of 2,000. Her spoken-word music CD, *Renaissance Woman/Race Woman*, a collaboration with musicians Ciro Hurtado and Kim Jordan, was released in 2001. Since 2006, Dr. Yancey has been a public health commentator for the Los Angeles National Public Radio affiliate, KPCC.

Index

24 Hour Fitness, 114
49ers, San Francisco, 204
5 a Day, 130, 131, 136

accelerometry, 6, 181, 189, 204
Action for Healthy Kids, 202, 249
active living, 12, 127
Active Living Research, 152, 181
advertising, 33; active lifestyles for the
    affluent, 109; early branding, 5; ethnically
    targeted, 125; exercise, 116; healthy life-
    style promotion, 128, 230, 234; limitations,
    9; stigma of healthy options, 74; targeting
    children, 4, 6; unhealthy lifestyle, 6,
    10–11, 92
advocacy, in physical activity promotion, 12,
    13, 20, 65, 67, 129, 151, 174, 212
aerobics, 85, 87

African American Collaborative Obesity
    Research Network (AACORN), 203
African Americans: attitudes toward activ-
    ity, 35; body image, 125; chronic disease
    rates, 198; culturally appropriate
    approaches, 147; culturally targeted mar-
    keting, 70, 71, 196; culture and values, 62,
    70, 88, 94, 100, 120, 149; culture as market-
    ing tool, 120, 125; gender roles, 39; health
    disparities, 42, 45, 128, 137, 170; health sta-
    tus perception, 38; history, 41, 117, 239;
    institutions and organizations, 203; mes-
    saging in media, 137; obesity prevalence,
    6; social expectations, 147; target of
    health-compromising advertising, 123;
    television habits, 35, 36
African dance, 98
Alzheimer's disease, 23, 55, 104, 107, 221

Amazon, 88, 234
American Cancer Society, 161
American College of Sports Medicine, 7, 95
American Heart Association, 67
American Indians. *See* Native Americans
American Journal of Preventive Medicine, 104
American Journal of Public Health, 216
An Old Soul with a Young Spirit, 92, 133, 134
Animal Trackers, 179
Asian, 2, 3, 149; gender roles, 35; mind-body practices, 62
Assiniboine Indians, 182
Association of Black Women Physicians, 126
AuYoung, Mona, 136

baby boomers, 24, 25, 138, 221, 234
Bally's, 116, 120
Banks, Tyra, 233
barriers to engaging in physical activity, 2, 3, 4, 32, 34, 35, 70, 76, 114, 141
basketball, 152, 209; as an adult, 17; as asset, 133; as a child, 17; at Northwestern, 78; as outlet, 17; in poetry, 44; recreation, 81, 104, 109, 149, 215; women in sports, 41–43, 43
Bastani, Roshan, 182
Battle Creek Sanitarium, 110
behavior change models: diffusion of innovations, 143, 222, 224, 225, 230; Meta-Volition Model, 222, 223, 226–28; social cognitive theory, 224, 225; social control theory, 98, 173, 220, 228
Berkeley Media Studies Center, 217
Bernert, Kristin, 215
Berrien, Todd, 92, 95, 125, 239
Best, Bobby, 171
Bidi Bidi Bom Bom, 188
Biggest Loser, 168
biking, 29, 57, 220, 235
Blair, Steve, 113
Blanks, Billy, 114
BMI, 23, 199, 201
body mass index. *See* BMI
Bonner, Deltra, 181
booster breaks, 180
Bracho, America, 148
Breslow, Lester, 84, 85, 87, 238
brief bouts of physical activity, 115, 180. *See also* short bouts
Broberg, Kelly, 210

Brown Miller Communications, 103
Brown v. Board of Education, 18
Brown, Helene, 52
Brownson, Ross, 52
Buch, Amy, 210
built environment, 4, 12, 19, 60, 129, 190, 220; influence on activity, 12, 59, 60, 235
Bush administration, 127
Bush, George H. W., 73
Bush, George W., 128

California Center for Public Health Advocacy, 237
California Contract Cities Association, 209
California Health Interview Survey, 202
Caltrans, 190
cancer: activity as prevention and treatment, 55; call to action, 62, 108, 161; control and prevention, 42, 56, 83, 84, 120, 180; economics, 4; funding policy, 221; inactivity as risk factor, 23; loss of productive years, 46; obesity as risk factor, 23; screening services, 83, 94; treatment and research centers, 88, 182
Cancer Prevention and Control Research Network, 182
cardiovascular disease, 67, 68, 75, 107, 108, 161, 235; activity as treatment, 55; call to action, 62; co-morbidity, 81
Cascade County, 182
Casey Family Programs, 148, 162
CDC: health promotion campaign, 127, 210; recommended activity guidelines, 4, 6–8, 95, 179, 194, 196; research and support, 129, 182, 197, 208, 237; statistics, 26, 29; work environment, 40
Center of Excellence in the Elimination of Disparities, 182, 214
Centers for Disease Control and Prevention. *See* CDC
Charles Drew University, 90, 91, 121
childhood obesity: etiology, 32; incidence and prevalence, 6, 24, 179, 221; philanthropic organizations, 202; prevention, 53, 58, 204, 212, 217; treatment, 67, 191, 202, 228, 237
cholesterol, 8, 56, 187, 198, 227
chronic disease: control, 53, 75, 129, 187, 222, 232, 236; epidemic, 118; increased risk, 91,

234, 238; prevention, 7, 8, 14, 15, 53-55; sedentariness as risk factor, 30
Chronic Disease Prevention and Health Promotion Division, 94, 187, 197
Clark, Maureen, 237
Clinton, Bill, 67, 73
cognitive benefits, of physical activity, 20, 67, 73, 150, 205, 230
cognitive dissonance, 101
Community Resource Project, 237
competition, 113, 119, 130, 142, 168, 187, 193, 214, 234
Cooper Institute for Aerobics Research, 85, 96, 113, 115
Cooper, Kenneth, 86-88, 113
Coordinated Approach to Child Health. See PASS & CATCH
Cordis de Mexico, 188
Costanza, Michael, 57
couch potatoes, 5, 142
Crystal Stairs, 164, 167-69
cultural assets, 62, 149
cultural competency or proficiency, 48
cultural resonance or salience, 149
cultural sensitivity, 42, 178
culture: clash between nutrition and exercise science, 74; definition, 47-48; inclusiveness, 70-71, 76; as marketing tool, 71, 84, 120, 196; and social norms, 62, sociocultural influences, 21, 74; targeted approaches, 47, 152, 170, 197; 149; and values, 62, 70, 88, 94, 100, 120
Curves, 111

Dairy Council, 234
dance: as cultural asset, 62; in *Instant Recess*, 14, 96, 123, 142, 183, 194, 206
Dance Dance Revolution, 112
Dante, 10
Delta Sigma Theta Sorority, 169-70
Department of Health and Human Services, 13
designated driver, 9
diabesity, 28
diabetes, 11, 221; activity as prevention and management, 55, 56; co-morbidity, 81, 83; diagnosis as catalyst to activity, 67; economics, 4, 25; epidemiology, 7, 24; family history, 161, 187; inactivity as risk factor,

23, 24, 221; loss of productive years, 46; obesity as risk factor, 187; philanthropic organizations, 202; rising mortality among youth, 221
Diaz, Reina, 209
Dietary Guidelines for Americans, 8
Discovery Channel, 162
Disney World, 191
disparities. *See* health disparities
dissemination of *Instant Recess*, 117, 162, 180-182, 220
Dodgers, Los Angeles, 214
DodgerVision, 214
Don Quixote, 79
Donnelly, Joe, 217
Dorfman, Lori, 40, 217
drinking and driving, 9, 173, 203, 228
Duarte, CA, 208
Duda, Catherine, 99
Duke University, 80, 82

Eastern European, 186
economics, of physical activity, 19, 32, 55-58, 72, 76, 173, 184, 189, 224
Eisenberg, Joni, 99
Energizers, 178, 179
energy imbalance, 59, 73
EnviroMedia, 25, 103
environmental change approaches, 47, 53, 156, 180
epidemiology, of physical activity, 3, 5, 6, 23, 42
equity, 113. *See also* health disparities
ER, 137
ESPN, 74, 183
evolutionary programming, 5, 6, 10, 27, 28, 62
exercise: definition, 5n1; mimetics, 54; physiology, 8, 47; prescription, 51, 218

Facebook, 148, 234
facilitators of physical activity participation, 3, 90, 120, 141-143
faith based approaches, 47, 51, 91, 92, 149, 170-72, 181, 208
Falcons, Atlanta, 202, 204
Felder, Donald, 162
Fenton, Mark, 224
Fielding, Jonathan, 96

Fighting Cancer with Fitness, 94, 116, 120, 126
Fitness *Funatics*, 121
FitnessGRAM, 115
FitWIC, 215
Fonda, Jane, 114
Food and Drug Administration, 73
food industry, 10, 19, 63–66, 68, 72, 109, 127
Food Politics, 18
Fork Union Military Academy, 133
Forsyth County, 205, 207
Fort Peck Reservation, 183
fountain of change, 224
Fourthmeal, Taco Bell, 11
FriarFit, San Diego Padres, 212–15
Friedman, Tom, 217

Galinsky, Traci, 185
Game Time Tour, 204
Gandhi, 238
Garcia, Byron, 192
Gaston-Greene, Lois, 208
Gen Xers, 25, 138, 221
Gen Yers, 221
gender equity, 35
gender issues, 35, 41, 114
gender roles, 46
General Foods, 123
Georgino, Donna, 208
Gold's Gym, 111
Goldmon, Moses, 171–72
Great Depression, 16, 117
Green, Larry, 52
Gulick Project, 98
gyms/fitness facilities, 7–8, 49; affordability, 4; barriers to use, 73, 144, 156, 161, 188; cultural sensitivity, 42; as incentive, 210; increasing usage, 69, 94, 97, 120, 125, 150, 156; privileges, 4, 114; recruitment stategies, 88; use in intervention study, 90, 94

Halfon, Neal, 82
Handler, Eric, 210
Harvard University, 11, 45, 60; Alcohol Project, 9; Nurses' Health Study, 56
Head Start, 179, 208
health disparities, 24, 34, 35, 37–38, 42, 45–46, 61, 114, 128, 137, 170
health effects, of physical activity, 8, 11, 87,

118, 143, 144, 190. *See also* cognitive benefits
health information, 10, 11; inadequacy in effecting behavior change, 9–11
Healthy Active Children Policy, 229
Healthy Eating Active Living, 128, 231, 237
healthy food policies, 153–54, 199
Healthy People objectives, 13
heart disease, 11, 23, 55, 56, 113, 120 ; activity as prevention, 55; loss of productive years, 46. *See also* cardiovascular disease
Heinen, LuAnn, 162
Hickey, Gordon, 132
historical perspectives on physical activity, 5, 86-88, 144
HIV, 47, 70, 122, 221
Hollywood, Health & Society project, 137
Hopkins, Jammie, 98
Horton, Mark, 210
Hot, Flat, and Crowded, 217
hypertension, 55; co-morbidity, 81, 83; economics, 4; family history, 187; obesity as risk factor, 187, 198

Imagineering, 191
incentives, 70, 121, 192
Institute of Medicine, 32, 109, 243, 245, 249
integrated approaches, 76, 77, 94, 163, 166, 176, 209
integration of physical activity into daily routine, 6, 7, 31, 61, 68, 76, 99, 209
Interfaith Pilgrimage of the Middle Passage, 238
International Life Sciences Institute, 96
Iowa Writers' Workshop, 132
Isaac, Fik, 188
Ishmael, Rocket, 145
Italian chefs stretching, 96
iTunes, 234

Jackson, Dick, 204
Jackson, Michael, 192
James, Harold, 134
Johnson & Johnson, 188
Johnson, Magic, 114
Jordan, Kim, 238
joy of movement, 14, 146

Kaiser Permanente, 128, 129, 180

Kessler, David, 73
knowledge, health, 49, 88, 137
Kohl, Bill, 96, 177
KPCC, 136
Kreuter, Matt, 132
Kumanyika, Shiriki, 35, 70

L. L. Bean, 122, 131, 135, 184, 216
Latinos: attitudes toward activity, 35; clini-
    cal treatment perspective, 18, culturally
    resonant or salient approaches, 147; cul-
    turally targeted marketing, 33, 71, 84, 196;
    culture and values, 48, 62, 100, 149; gender
    roles, 35, 39; health disparities, 45; health
    status perception, 38; intra-cultural differ-
    ences, 139; obesity prevalence, 6; South
    American, 186
leisure time physical activity, 8, 30, 87, 113,
    114
Leslie, Joanne, 94
Let's Move initiative, 136
Levine, Jim, 99
Lift Off!: adaptability, 98, 201, 203; adoption,
    153, 170, 181, 182, 202, 210; concept, 96, 194;
    design for all levels of fitness, 194; devel-
    opment, 211; dissemination, 96, 99, 125,
    148, 171, 208; evaluation, 124; events
    around, 211; evolution, 124; implementa-
    tion, 166; integration, 196, 197, 211; inter-
    vention, 176, 194; original video, 187;
    return on investment, 126; similar inter-
    ventions, 178; the right messenger, 138;
    similar programs, 96
Live for Life, 188
Los Angeles County Department of Public
    Health, 38, 124, 176, 197, 203, 215
Los Angeles Stars, 203
Los Angeles Times, 88, 132
Los Angeles Unified School District, 67
Los Angeles Urban League, 152
Love, Susan, 88

MADD, 9
Madonna, 114
Maibach, Ed, 118
Maine, 184
Making the Grade with Diet and Exercise, 178
March Madness, 74
Marcus, Bess, 71

marketing, 33, 66, 108, 109, 113, 119, 121, 127.
    See also social marketing
Maternal, Child, and Adolescent Health
    Program, 165–67
Maugham, Somerset, 48
Mavericks, Dallas, 202
Mayo Clinic, 31, 100
McCarthy, Bill, 49, 84, 94
McDaniel-Lowe, Sharon, 148
McDonald's, 32, 77, 125
Mead, Margaret, 238
media representation of physical activity, 1,
    13, 36, 46, 110, 113–115
Medicaid, 82, 233
Medicare, 25, 233
meta-volition, 224
Mexican Ministry of Health, 96, 176
Milbank Boys and Girls Club, 145
Miles, Octavia, 88, 90, 94, 120, 161
Miller Brewing Co., 92
Milton Jones, DeLisha, 215
Minds at Play, 191
Mitchell, Dan, 192
MLBFit, 214
Montana State University, 182
Morabia, Alfredo, 57
Mothers Against Drunk Driving. See MADD
motivational interviewing, 47
mouse potatoes, 5, 112, 142, 191. See also sed-
    entary behavior
Move and Make It Matter, 188
Moving with Tradition, 183
My Gym, 111

National Business Group on Health, 162
National Health Club Association, 116
National Institutes of Health, 162, 183, 199
National Physical Activity Plan, 71, 118, 237
National Women's Law Center, 45
Native Americans, 35, 62, 149
NBA, 41, 43, 114, 202
Neel, Joe, 134
Neighmond, Patti, 134
Nestle, Marion, 18
Network for a Healthy California, 237
New Aerobics, The, 87
New England Journal of Medicine, 121
New York Times, 217
New York Times Magazine, 42

NFL, 202, 234
Nielsen, Brigitte, 114
Northern California Bay Bridge project, 162
Northwestern University, 78
NPR, 134, 136, 138, 183, 192
Nutrition Network, 208

Obama administration, 117, 127, 221
Obama, Barack, 182, 219, 238
Obama, Michelle, 136
obesity: activity as prevention, 15, 55–59, 73,
    129, 150, 221; and advertising, 33; as bar-
    rier to activity, 140, 141, 145; chronic dis-
    ease risk factor, 46, 68, 118, 187; control
    and prevention, 18, 66, 75, 76, 222; defini-
    tion, 23; diversions from the problem, 31;
    economics, 4, 25, 55, 58, 221; epidemiology,
    2, 6, 23, 58, 65, 219, 231; evolutionary biol-
    ogy governing, 12, 27–28; framing of
    problem, 40; genetic disposition, 39;
    health campaigns, 47, 170, 204; health dis-
    parities, 36; health disparity risk factor,
    24; and inactivity, 23; as inactivity risk
    factor, 23, 30; limits of exercise-only
    approach, 65; limits of nutrition-only
    approach, 32, 49; long-term effects, 23;
    morbidity and mortality, 11, 23; need for
    large scale solutions, 13, 217; personal
    responsibility, 49; physiology, 8; policy
    advocacy, 65–69, 73, 74, 125; politics, 39,
    66–68; prevention strategy, 63, 76, 121, 136,
    204; and sedentariness, 31; social and per-
    sonal toll, 25; stigma, 10, 27, 36, 40. See also
    overweight
obesogenic society, 46, 73, 74, 144
occupational safety, 122
Olshansky, Jay, 121
Orange County Health Care Agency, 182,
    210, 211
organizational adoption 124, 125, 179, 182,
    185, 198; approaches, 90, 100; implementa-
    tion, 12, 14, 151–55, 163–72
Orion, Dean, 191
Overton, Jeff, 215
overweight, 10, 31, 35, 111; among role mod-
    els and peers, 36; body image, 125; defini-
    tion, 23, 246; economics, 26, 55; epidemiol-
    ogy, 6, 23, 24, 26, 198; health campaigns,

147, 194; health status perception, 38, 39;
    media portrayal of minorities, 36, 137;
    messengers and messaging, 38, 196; moti-
    vation, 96, 100; recruitment and retention,
    42, 58. See also obesity

Pacific Islanders, 149
Pacifica Radio Network, 99, 134, 237
Pad Squad, 212
Padres, San Diego, 66, 205, 212, 214, 215
Paltrow, Gwyneth, 114
Paris, 79, 80
Parker, Candace, 215
Partnership for a Healthier America, 136
PASS & CATCH, 178, 180
Pausa para tu Salud, 96, 176
PBS, 138
pedometer, 6, 91, 123, 170, 189
peer pressure and influences, 3, 61, 69, 98,
    142, 173. See also social influences
philanthropy, 230
Physical Activity Across the Curriculum,
    178, 217
Physical Activity Guidelines for Americans,
    8, 117, 118
Physical Activity Liaison to my Sisters, 170
physical education, 33, 34, 66, 67, 69, 72, 122,
    177, 178, 205, 229
physical environment, 61, 62, 236
physical inactivity, 25, 26, 57, 58, 70, 189, 221,
    233; energy imbalance, 23; increased dis-
    ease risk, 23, 45; need for intervention, 96,
    226; physiology, 8, 226; poor health status
    and outcomes, 24, 52, 176; population bur-
    den, 6, 21, 71; prevalence in schools, 33;
    relationship to perceived weight, 38;
    social engineering, 29. See also sedentary
    behavior
Pioneering Innovation Award, 129
Pixar, 1
poems: Ain' Like There's Hunger, 102–3; Blue
    Grease, 37; Did You Ever Have a Mentor?, 86;
    In My Father's House, 239; Recapturing
    Recess, 15; She Went Away, 105–6; We, Too,
    Are Ballas, 44; Wilma Rudolph's Legacy, 240
policy and environmental change, 68, 69,
    143, 232. See also environmental change
    approaches

politics, 75
Pollan, Michael, 160
Principles of Engagement for Long-Term
    Success, 202, 204, 214
Professional Athletes Council, 137, 143, 202–
    4, 214
program champion, 91, 124, 168, 187, 189
Project LEAN, 212
promoting physical activity, 9, 67, 76, 110,
    112, 212, 220
Pronk, Nico, 154
protective factor, 56–58, 68
public health infrastructure, 76
Public Health Institute, 176
push strategies, 190; adoption, 223; evalua
    tion, 164; favoring at risk populations, 191;
    healthy choice as easy choice, 15, 20, 71,
    173; obligatory v. nonobligatory, 28, 76;
    occupational safety, 188; paid company
    time, 125, 200; rationale, 222

Rabe, John, 136
Racial and Ethnic Approaches to Commu-
    nity Health, 197, 198
Recess Before Lunch, 179
recess model: adoption, 148, 164; as push
    strategy, 173, 191; captive audience, 169;
    conflict, 168; consistency with national
    values, 193; cost-effectiveness, 217; diffu-
    sion, 180; ease of adoption, 218; effective-
    ness, 194; element of fun, 122; evaluation,
    175; factors influencing activity, 100; fit-
    ness vs weight loss, 146; influence on
    sociocultural environment, 98; institu-
    tional support, 199; institutional support,
    182; level of investment, 216; origins, 81;
    proliferation, 177; promotion, 137; similar
    interventions, 178; target audience, 169;
    Ten Commandments, 143
Releford, Bill, 121
Replacements, Ltd, 186
return on investment, 58, 130, 136, 184, 186
Reuters, 136
Richmond Times Dispatch, 30, 132
Roan, Shari, 132
Robert Wood Johnson Foundation, 60, 152,
    171, 181, 207
Robinson, Konnie, 181

Rock! Richmond, 91, 92
role models, 36, 40, 53, 82, 146, 201, 202, 225
Rossum, Allen, 202–5
Russell, Jane, 110

Saatchi & Saatchi, 92
¡Sabor y Energía!, 124
Safe Routes to Schools, 60
safety, 35, 36, 66, 122, 148, 155, 185–189, 210,
    211, 236
Sallis, Jim, 152
San Diego State University, 152
Satcher, David, 76
Saturday Night Live, 234
Sawyer, Carolyn, 205
scalability, 13, 27, 71, 76, 129, 143, 222
sedentary behavior: and academic decline,
    151; bad for business, 184; discouraging,
    12, 56, 98, 194, 228, 235, 236; economic
    costs, 4, 25, 57, 58, 189; energy expended,
    190; entertainment, 36, 112; epidemic, 2,
    58, 219; fitness status, 176; and formerly
    fit, 146; gender diferences, 37; health dis-
    parities, 34; health status, 125; impact of
    small changes, 191; incentivizing change,
    210; individual problem, 2; industry pro-
    motion, 32; intervention, 13, 95, 99, 100,
    126, 145, 191, 197; later years, 104; long-
    term effects, 23; marketing, 6, 31, 40; mobi-
    lization, 112; morbidity and mortality, 23;
    negative spiral, 35; obesity escalation, 65;
    overcoming desire to be active, 141; perva-
    siveness, 2, 35, 56, 57; poor outcomes, 58;
    promoting products, 130; regulation to
    decrease, 235; reverting back to, 171; social
    impact, 52, 220; societal problem, 2; statis-
    tics, 6, 22, 198, 200; strategies to eliminate,
    75; threat to social infrastructure, 24;
    video games, 75; and youth, 179
sedentary suicide, 69
Self-Esteem through Creative Expression Defy-
    ing Expectations (SECEDE), 134
Seventh Day Adventists, 110
Shaw University Divinity School, 171
short bouts of physical activity, 12, 56, 57,
    70, 124, 134-136, 145, 193. See also brief
    bouts
shrinking mirror syndrome, 161

Simmons, Richard, 3, 114
Sioux Indians, 182
sitting, 15, 33, 235, 236; prolonged periods, 7, 23, 59, 113, 123, 135, 152, 160, 172, 203, 235
Small Steps, 115
smoke-free workplace act, 69, 238
smoking, 23, 81, 98, 185, 202, 203, 231, 238
Snow, Michelle, 44
Soap Box, 192
Sobero, Raúl, 210
social environment, 9, 60, 62
social marketing: basis for *Instant Recess*, 96, 124; curbing drinking and driving, 10; difference from commercial marketing, 109; early activity messaging, 113; health campaigns, 91, 115, 119-121, 127-129; physical activity examples, 119; promotion of, 115; tailored messaging, 100, 147; within health departments, 92, 95
social norms, 39, 51, 98, 100. *See also* culture
sociocultural environment, 62. *See also* culture
Sony Eye Toy, 112
spark plugs, 217, 226
SparKids, 215
SPARKing Motion, 214, 215
Sparks, Los Angeles, 214, 215
sports and fitness industry alliances, 230
Sports Are Good for Girls, 30
Sprint, 191
St. John's Christian Methodist Episcopal (CME), 171–72, 181
Stackhouse, Jerry, 202
Staples Center, 215
State Children's Health Insurance Program, 53
Story Road Films, 182
Streeter, Oscar, 50
stroke, 23, 46, 55, 56, 107, 108. *See also* cardiovascular disease
Subirats, Elena, 96
Super Bowl, 205, 234
Sweatin' with the Oldies, 3

Taco Bell, 11
Take 10!, 96, 177, 178, 179
Tapia, Roberto, 176
Taylor, Clinton (Junior), 205
Taylor, Wendell, 180

technological influences, 5, 28-29, 115, 148, 149, 152
Teen Activity Project, 123
Telephone Bar and Grill, 134
television: and activity, 31; healthy lifestyle programming, 110; messages, 128, 129, 137, 212, 231; and obesity, 30, 36; sedentary behavior, 4, 6, 117, 141, 142, 200; teens' watching habits, 35
Thompson, Tina, 215
Thriller, 152, 192
Thrive, Kaiser Permanente, 128–29
Thurston, Rebecca, 133
Title IX, 42, 44, 45, 113
tobacco control, 69, 94, 122, 136, 194, 222, 237; lessons from anti-tobacco campaign, 9–15, 52, 59, 122, 143, 228
top-down strategies, 12, 40, 118
Tubman, Harriet, 238
Tufts, Susan, 131, 185

UCLA: professional career, 18, 83; research study, 116, 152, 164–71, 182, 201, 208, 225; research team, 9, 33, 38, 163, 190, 199, 212
UCLA Kaiser Permanente Center for Health Equity, 180
Ugly Betty, 46
Underground Railroad, 238
Union Chapel Baptist Church, 181
University of California at San Francisco, 52
University of Kansas, 178, 217
University of Pennsylvania, 68, 70, 203
University of Southern California, 137
University of Texas, 180
upstream approaches, 51
urban planning, 68
US Department of Agriculture (USDA), 124, 127, 237
Usher, 234

VERB, 127, 128
video games: physical or active, 75, 112; sedentary, 4, 32, 33, 40, 130, 203
Vietnam War, 87
Vogue, 79

Wake Forest University, 181
walking, 7, 56, 137; daily routine, 4, 12, 190, 209; groups, 51, 76, 91, 146, 170, 186, 189;

meetings, 15, 125, 135, 148, 153, 156, 163, 226; for recreation, 3, 12, 45, 108, 140, 150, 154, 235; for transportation, 29, 129, 191
WALL-E, 1
Washington University, 52, 132
Washington, DC, 237
Watson, Diane, 90
WBAI, 134
weight control, 3, 19, 55, 73, 74, 75
weight loss, 27, 46, 116, 125, 146, 168, 233
Weight of the Nation, 129
Weismuller, Johnny, 110
Wellness Warrior, 124
Western Health Reform Institute, 110
Westinghouse, 188
White House, 69, 81, 136
whites, 7, 24, 35, 186; and advertising, 33, 71; and being thin, 3; body image, 38; cultural targeting, 149; role models, 202; television habits, 36
Whitt-Glover, Melicia, 171, 207

Whittier Health Center, 164–65
WIC (Women, Infants, and Children), 208, 215, 216, 237
WIC Walks the Talk, 215, 216
Wii Fit, 112
Williams, Serena, 46
Williams, Venus, 46
Wilson, Shawn, 202
Winfrey, Oprah, 114, 233
Winston-Salem, 171, 205, 207, 208
WNBA, 42, 43, 78, 214
WORKING (Working Out Regularly Keeps Individuals Nurtured and Going), 199
worksite wellness, 152, 164–169, 185, 216
World War II, 16, 85
WPFW, 99, 237

YMCA, 62, 98, 99, 111
YouTube, 152, 192, 234

Zimmerman, Fred, 237

Text: 10/14 Palatino, 9/14 Univers Light
Display: Bauer Bodoni, Univers Light Condensed
Compositor: BookMatters, Berkeley
Printer: Sheridan Books, Inc.